*Quick*FACTS™

Colon
CANCER

What You Need to Know—NOW

Books published by the American Cancer Society

A Breast Cancer Journey: Your Personal Guidebook, Second Edition

American Cancer Society Consumers Guide to Cancer Drugs, Second Edition, Wilkes, Ades, and Krakoff

American Cancer Society's Complete Guide to Colorectal Cancer, Levin et al.

American Cancer Society's Complete Guide to Prostate Cancer, Bostwick et al.

American Cancer Society's Guide to Pain Control, Revised Edition

Angels & Monsters: A child's eye view of cancer, Murray and Howard

Because... Someone I Love Has Cancer: Kids' Activity Book

Cancer in the Family: Helping Children Cope with a Parent's Illness, Heiney et al.

Cancer: What Causes It, What Doesn't

Caregiving: A Step-By-Step Resource for Caring for the Person with Cancer at Home, Revised Edition, Houts and Bucher

Coming to Terms with Cancer: A Glossary of Cancer-Related Terms, Laughlin

Couples Confronting Cancer: Keeping Your Relationship Strong, Fincannon and Bruss

Crossing Divides: A Couple's Story of Cancer, Hope, and Hiking Montana's Continental Divide, Bischke

Eating Well, Staying Well During and After Cancer, Bloch et al.

Good for You! Reducing Your Risk of Developing Cancer

Healthy Me: A Read-along Coloring & Activity Book, Hawthorne (illustrated by Blyth)

Informed Decisions: The Complete Book of Cancer Diagnosis, Treatment, and Recovery, Second Edition, Eyre, Lange, and Morris

Kicking Butts: Quit Smoking and Take Charge of Your Health

Lymphedema: Understanding and Managing Lymphedema After Cancer Treatment

Our Mom Has Cancer, Ackermann and Ackermann

When the Focus Is on Care: Palliative Care and Cancer, Foley et al.

Also by the American Cancer Society

American Cancer Society's Healthy Eating Cookbook: A celebration of food, friends, and healthy living, Third Edition

Celebrate! Healthy Entertaining for Any Occasion

Kids' First Cookbook: Delicious-Nutritious Treats to Make Yourself!

QuickFACTS™

From the Experts at the American Cancer Society

Colon CANCER

What You Need to Know—NOW

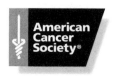

Published by American Cancer Society / Health Promotions
1599 Clifton Road NE, Atlanta, Georgia 30329, USA

Printed in the United States of America
Cover designed by Jill Dible, Atlanta, GA

5 4 3 2 1   06 07 08 09 10

Library of Congress Cataloging-in-Publication Data
Quick facts colon cancer : what you need to know—now /
from the experts at the American Cancer Society.
    p. cm.
 ISBN-13: 978-0-944235-67-6 (pbk. : alk. paper)
 ISBN-10: 0-944235-67-0 (pbk.)
1. Colon (Anatomy)—Cancer—Popular works. I. American Cancer Society.

 RC280.C6Q53 2007
 616.99'4347—dc22

                                    2006016960

A Note to the Reader

This information represents the views of the doctors and nurses serving on the American Cancer Society's Cancer Information Database Editorial Board. These views are based on their interpretation of studies published in medical journals, as well as their own professional experience.

The treatment information in this document is not official policy of the Society and is not intended as medical advice to replace the expertise and judgment of your cancer care team. It is intended to help you and your family make informed decisions, together with your doctor.

Your doctor may have reasons for suggesting a treatment plan different from these general treatment options. Don't hesitate to ask him or her questions about your treatment options.

 For more information, contact your American Cancer Society at 800-ACS-2345 or http://www.cancer.org

Table of Contents

Treatments

Questions To Ask

After Treatment

Latest Research

Resources

Dictionary

Index

Your Colorectal Cancer

What Is Cancer?

Cancer* develops when cells in a part of the body begin to grow out of control. Although there are many kinds of cancer, they all start because of out-of-control growth of abnormal cells.

Normal body cells grow, divide, and die in an orderly fashion. During the early years of a person's life, normal cells divide more rapidly until the person becomes an adult. After that, cells in most parts of the body divide only to replace worn-out or dying cells and to repair injuries.

Because cancer cells continue to grow and divide, they are different from normal cells. Instead of dying, they outlive normal cells and continue to form new abnormal cells.

Cancer cells can sometimes travel to other parts of the body where they begin to grow and replace normal tissue. This process, called **metastasis**, occurs as the cancer cells get into the bloodstream or lymph vessels of our body. When cells from a cancer like colorectal cancer spread to another organ like the liver, the cancer is still called colorectal cancer, not liver cancer.

* Terms in **bold type** are further explained in the dictionary that begins on page 99.

Cancer cells develop because of damage to **DNA**. This substance is in every cell and directs all activities. Most of the time when DNA becomes damaged the body is able to repair it. In cancer cells, the damaged DNA is not repaired. People can inherit damaged DNA, which accounts for inherited cancers. More often, though, a person's DNA becomes damaged by exposure to something in the environment, like smoking.

Cancer usually forms as a tumor. Some cancers, like leukemia, do not form tumors. Instead, these cancer cells involve the blood and blood-forming organs and circulate through other tissues where they grow.

Remember that not all tumors are cancerous. **Benign** (non-cancerous) tumors do not spread to other parts of the body (metastasize) and, with rare exceptions, are not life threatening.

Different types of cancer can behave very differently. For example, lung cancer and breast cancer are very different diseases. They grow at different rates and respond to different treatments. That is why people with cancer need treatment that is aimed at their particular kind of cancer.

Cancer is the second leading cause of death in the United States. Nearly half of all men and a little over one third of all women in the United States will develop cancer during their lifetimes. Today, millions of people are living with cancer or have had cancer. The risk of developing most types of cancer can be reduced by changes in a person's lifestyle—for example, by quitting smoking, eating a better diet, and increasing physical activity. The sooner a cancer is found and treatment begins, the better are the chances for living for many years.

What Is Colorectal Cancer?

Colorectal cancer is a term used to refer to cancer that develops in the colon or the rectum. The colon and rectum are parts of the digestive system, which is also called the gastrointestinal, or GI, system. The digestive system processes food for energy and rids the body of solid waste matter (fecal matter or stool).

After food is chewed and swallowed, it travels through the esophagus to the stomach. There it is partly broken down and then sent to the **small intestine**, also known as the **small bowel**. The word "small" refers to the diameter of the small intestine, which is narrower than that of the large bowel. Actually, the small intestine is the longest segment of the digestive system—about 20 feet. The small intestine continues breaking down the food and absorbs most of the nutrients. The small bowel joins the colon in the right lower abdomen. The **colon** (also called the **large bowel** or **large intestine**) is a muscular tube about 5 feet long. The colon continues to absorb water and mineral nutrients from the food matter and serves as a storage place for waste matter. The waste matter left after this process is feces and goes into the **rectum**, the final 6 inches of the digestive system. From there it passes out of the body through the **anus**.

The colon has 4 sections:

- The first section is called the **ascending colon**. It begins where the small bowel attaches to the colon and extends upward on the right side of the abdomen.
- The second section is called the **transverse colon** since it goes across the body from the right to the left side in the upper abdomen.

- The third section, the **descending colon**, continues downward on the left side.
- The fourth section is known as the **sigmoid colon** because of its "S" or "sigmoid" shape. The sigmoid colon joins the rectum, which in turn joins the anus, or the opening where waste (fecal) matter passes out of the body.

The wall of each of these sections of the colon and rectum has several layers of tissue. Colorectal cancer starts in the innermost layer and can grow through some or all of the other layers. Knowing a little about these layers is important, because the **stage** (extent of spread) of a colorectal cancer depends to a great degree on how deeply it invades into these layers.

Colon cancer and rectal cancer, collectively known as colorectal cancer, have many features in common.

In most people, colorectal cancers develop slowly over a period of several years. Before a true cancer develops, a growth of tissue or tumor usually begins as a non-cancerous polyp, which may eventually change into cancer. A polyp develops on the lining of the colon or rectum. Certain kinds of polyps, called **adenomatous polyps** or **adenomas**, are types that have the potential to become cancerous.

There are other kinds of polyps called *hyperplastic* and *inflammatory* polyps. Inflammatory polyps and hyperplastic polyps, in general, are not considered pre-cancerous. But some doctors think that some hyperplastic polyps might be pre-cancerous or a sign that the person may be more likely to develop adenomatous polyps and cancer, particularly if they grow in the right or ascending colon. Another kind of pre-cancerous condition is called **dysplasia**. This is usually seen in people with diseases, such as ulcerative colitis or Crohn's colitis, which cause chronic inflammation of the colon.

Once cancer forms within a polyp, it can eventually begin to grow into the wall of the colon or rectum. Once they are in the wall, the cancer cells can grow into blood vessels or lymph vessels. Lymph vessels are thin, tiny channels that carry away waste and fluid. They first drain into nearby lymph nodes, which are bean-shaped structures that help fight against infections. When they spread into blood vessels, the cancer cells can travel to distant parts of the body. This process of spread is called **metastasis**.

More than 95% of colorectal cancers are **adeno-carcinomas**. These are cancers of the glandular cells that line the inside layer of the wall of the colon and rectum. Other less common types of tumors may also develop in the colon and rectum, such as:

- **carcinoid tumors**—these tumors develop from specialized hormone-producing cells of the intestine.
- **gastrointestinal stromal tumors**—these tumors develop from specialized cells in the wall of the colon called the "interstitial cells of Cajal." Some are benign (non-cancerous); others are malignant (cancerous). Although these cancers can be found anywhere in the gastrointestinal tract, they are unusual in the colon.
- **lymphomas**—these are cancers of immune system cells that typically develop in lymph nodes but also may start in the colon and rectum or other organs.

These more rare types of tumors are not covered in this document. Separate documents about gastrointestinal (digestive system) carcinoid and stromal tumors are available from the American Cancer Society. Information on lymphomas of the digestive system is included in the American Cancer Society document on non-Hodgkin lymphoma.

What Are the Key Statistics About Colorectal Cancer?

Excluding skin cancers, colorectal cancer is the third most common cancer diagnosed in men and in women in the United States. The American Cancer Society estimates that about 148,610 new cases of colorectal cancer (72,800 men and 75,810 women) will be diagnosed in 2006.

Colorectal cancer is the second leading cause of cancer-related deaths in the United States and is expected to cause about 55,170 deaths (27,870 men and 27,300 women) during 2006.

The death rate from colorectal cancer has been dropping for the past 15 years. There are a number of likely reasons for this. One reason is probably because polyps are being found by screening before they can develop into cancers. Also, colorectal cancer is being found earlier when it is easier to cure, and treatments have improved. Because of this, there are around 1 million survivors of colorectal cancer in the United States.

The **5-year relative survival rate** for people whose colorectal cancer is treated in an early stage, before it has spread, is greater than 90%. But only 39% of colorectal cancers are found at that early stage. Once the cancer has spread to nearby organs or lymph nodes, the 5-year relative survival rate goes down, and if cancer has spread to distant organs (i.e., the liver or lung) the 5-year survival is less than 10%.

The 5-year survival rate refers to the percentage of patients who live at least 5 years after their cancer is diagnosed. Many of these patients live much longer than 5 years after diagnosis. But the 5-year survival rate is used to produce a standard way of discussing **prognosis** (outlook). Five-year relative survival rates don't include patients dying of other diseases. Five-year relative survival rates are considered to be a more accurate way to describe the prognosis for patients with a particular type and stage of cancer. Of course, 5-year rates are based on patients diagnosed and first treated more than 5 years ago. These statistics may no longer be very accurate because improvements in treatment may result in a better outlook for more recently diagnosed patients.

Risk Factors and Causes

What Are the Risk Factors for Colorectal Cancer?

A **risk factor** is anything that increases your chance of getting a disease such as cancer. Different cancers have different risk factors. For example, unprotected exposure to strong sunlight is a risk factor for skin cancer, and smoking is a risk factor for cancers of the lungs, larynx, mouth, throat, esophagus, kidneys, bladder, colon, and several other organs. Researchers have identified several risk factors that increase a person's chance of developing colorectal polyps or colorectal cancer.

Age

While younger adults can develop colorectal cancer, your chances of developing colorectal cancer increase markedly after age 50. More than 90% of people diagnosed with colorectal cancer are older than 50.

A personal history of colorectal cancer

If you have had colorectal cancer, even though it has been completely removed, you are more likely to develop new cancers in other areas of the colon and rectum. The chances of this happening are greater if you had your first colorectal cancer when you were age 60 or younger.

A personal history of colorectal polyps

If you have had an adenomatous-type polyp, you are at increased risk of developing colorectal cancer. This is especially true if the polyps are large or if there are many of them.

A personal history of chronic inflammatory bowel disease

Chronic inflammatory bowel disease (IBD), including **ulcerative colitis** and **Crohn's disease**, is a condition in which the colon is inflamed over a long period of time. If you have chronic inflammatory bowel disease, your risk of developing colorectal cancer is increased. You should start being screened by colonoscopy 8 to 12 years after you were first diagnosed with IBD and testing should be repeated frequently (every 1 to 2 years). Often the first sign that cancer may be developing is called **dysplasia**. Dysplasia is a term that refers to cells that are no longer normal but they are not cancer yet. Inflammatory bowel disease is different than **irritable bowel syndrome (IBS),** which does not carry an increased risk for colorectal cancer.

A family history of colorectal cancer

Some cancers can "run in the family" because something in the environment has contributed to the development of cancer and/or because certain family members were born with, or inherited, an increased genetic susceptibility to cancer. While most colorectal cancers occur in people without a family history of colorectal cancer, those with a family history of colorectal cancer or adenomatous polyps in any first-degree relative younger than age 60, or in 2 or more first-degree relatives at any age are considered at increased risk for the disease. (First-degree relatives are defined as parents, siblings, and children.)

Familial disease

About 30% of people who develop colorectal cancer have disease that is familial. People who have a strong family history of colorectal cancer (as defined above), especially if the relatives are affected before the age of 60, are considered at increased risk of developing this disease. People with a family history of colorectal cancer need to talk with their doctor about beginning colorectal cancer testing at a younger age than age 50.

Inherited disease

About another 10% of people who develop colorectal cancer have an inherited genetic susceptibility to the disease. Approximately 3% to 5% of colorectal cancers are associated with the inherited colorectal cancer syndrome, called **hereditary non-polyposis colorectal cancer** (HNPCC), or **Lynch syndrome**. Another 1% of colorectal cancer cases are associated with the inherited syndrome, called **familial adenomatous polyposis** (FAP).

Familial adenomatous polyposis (FAP) is a disease where people typically develop hundreds of polyps in their colon and rectum. Usually this occurs between the ages of 5 and 40. Cancer usually develops in 1 or more of these polyps beginning at age 20. By age 40, almost all people with this disorder will have developed cancer if preventive surgery is not done. FAP is sometimes associated with Gardner syndrome, a condition that involves benign (non-cancerous) tumors of the skin, soft connective tissue, and bones. About 1% of all colorectal cancers are due to FAP.

Hereditary nonpolyposis colon cancer (HNPCC) is another clearly defined genetic syndrome. It accounts for 3% to 5% of all colorectal cancers. This syndrome also develops when people are relatively young. These people have polyps, but they only have a few, not hundreds as in FAP. Women with this condition also have a very high risk of developing cancer of the endometrium (lining of the upper part of the uterus). Other cancers associated with HNPCC include cancer of the ovary, stomach, small bowel, pancreas, kidney, ureters (tubes that carry urine from the kidneys to the bladder), and bile duct.

Doctors have found that most families with HNPCC have certain characteristics:

- At least 3 relatives have colorectal cancer.
- Two successive generations are involved.
- At least 1 relative had their cancer when they were younger than age 50.
- At least 2 of the people are first-degree relatives.

These are called the **Amsterdam criteria**. If any of these hold true for your family, then you might want to seek genetic counseling. But even if your family history satisfies the Amsterdam criteria, it doesn't mean you have HNPCC. Only about 60% of families who have the Amsterdam criteria have HNPCC. The other 40% do not; and although their colorectal cancer rate is higher than normal (about 2 times), it is not as high as that of people with HNPCC (about 6 times).

A second set of criteria for HNPCC, which has been recently revised, is called the **Bethesda criteria**. These are used to determine whether persons with colorectal cancer should have their cancer tested for genetic changes called microsatellite instability (MSI). These criteria include at least one of the following:

- The person is younger than 50 years.
- The person has or had another cancer (endometrial, stomach, pancreas, ovary, kidney or ureters, bile duct) that is associated with HNPCC.
- The person is younger than 60 years and the cancer has certain characteristics seen with MSI when viewed under the microscope.
- A first-degree relative has been diagnosed with a non-colorectal cancer often seen in HNPCC carriers (endometrial, stomach, pancreas, ovary, kidney, ureters, or bile duct) and is younger than 50 years.
- The person has 2 or more second-degree relatives who had an HNPCC-related tumor at any age.

MSI testing is the first step in laboratory testing to identify people with HNPCC. If a patient meets Bethesda criteria and has a tumor with MSI, more genetic testing will be needed to confirm that there is a mutation of one of the HNPCC genes. Still, the majority of people who meet the Bethesda criteria do not have HNPCC. On the other hand, about 2% of people with colorectal cancer who do not meet any of these criteria still have HNPCC when they are tested.

Doctors should also be suspicious of HNPCC if, instead of colorectal cancer, the family members have other cancers associated with this gene mutation. These are endometrial cancers, ovarian cancers, small bowel cancers, or cancer of the lining of the kidney or the ureters. Still, 1 family member younger than age 50 must have been diagnosed with colorectal cancer before a diagnosis of HNPCC is considered.

Accurate identification of families with these inherited syndromes is important. Then doctors can recommend specific measures, such as screening and other preventive measures, at an early age. Because several types of cancer can be associated with inherited colorectal cancer syndromes, all people should check their family medical history for polyps or any type of cancer. Those who develop polyps or cancer should inform other family members. People with a family history of colorectal polyps or cancer should consider genetic counseling, to review their family medical tree and determine whether genetic testing may be right for them. This will help them to make decisions about getting screened and treated at an early age.

Ethnic background

Jews of Eastern European descent (Ashkenazi Jews) have a higher rate of colorectal cancer. Recent research has found a genetic mutation leading to colorectal cancer in this group. This DNA change is present in about 6% of American Jews. In one study, about 10% of colorectal cancers in Jews of Eastern European descent were associated with this mutation. This gene change is called the I1307K APC mutation. It isn't clear, though, that this genetic change is responsible for the increased number of colorectal cancers in Ashkenazi Jews.

A diet mostly from animal sources

A diet that is high in fat, especially fats from animal sources, can increase your risk of colorectal cancer. Over time, eating a lot of red meats and processed meats can increase colorectal cancer risk. The American Cancer Society recommends choosing most of your foods from plant sources and limiting your intake of high-fat foods such as those from animal sources. The American Cancer Society also recommends eating at least 5 servings of fruits and vegetables every day and several servings of other foods from plant sources, such as breads, cereals, grain products, rice, pasta, or beans. Many fruits and vegetables contain substances that interfere with the process of cancer formation.

Physical inactivity

If you are not physically active, you have a greater chance of developing colorectal cancer.

Obesity

If you are very overweight, your risk of dying from colorectal cancer is increased.

Smoking

Recent studies indicate that smokers are 30% to 40% more likely than non-smokers to die of colorectal cancer. Smoking may be responsible for causing about 12% of fatal colorectal cancers. Almost everyone knows that smoking causes cancers in sites in the body that come in direct contact with the smoke, such as the mouth, larynx, and lungs. However, some of the cancer-causing substances are swallowed and can cause digestive system cancers, such as esophageal and colorectal cancer. Some of these substances are also absorbed into the bloodstream and can increase the risk of developing cancers of the kidneys, bladder, cervix, and other organs.

Alcohol intake

Colorectal cancer has been linked to the heavy use of alcohol. While some of this may be due to the effects of alcohol on folic acid in the body, it still would be wise to avoid heavy alcohol use.

Factors with Uncertain, Controversial, or Unproven Effects on Colorectal Cancer

Race

African Americans have the highest incidence and mortality. The reason for this is uncertain.

Diabetes

People with diabetes have a 30% to 40% increased chance of developing colorectal cancer. They also tend to have a higher death rate after diagnosis.

Night-shift work

Results of one single study suggest working a night shift at least 3 nights a month for at least 15 years may increase the risk of colorectal cancer in women. The study authors suggested this might be due to changes in melatonin (a hormone that responds to changes in light) levels in the body. More research is needed to confirm or refute this finding, however.

Other cancers and their treatment

A recent report on **testicular cancer** survivors found that these men had a higher rate of colorectal cancer. Men who receive **radiation therapy for prostate cancer** have been reported to have a higher risk of rectal cancer.

The American Cancer Society and several other medical organizations recommend earlier screening for people with increased colorectal cancer risk. These recommendations differ from those generally recommended for people at average risk. For more information, speak with your doctor and refer to the table in the "Can Colorectal Cancer Be Found Early?" (see page 30).

Do We Know What Causes Colorectal Cancer?

Although we do not know the exact cause of most colorectal cancers, there are certain known risk factors, and there is a great deal of research going on to find answers to the question.

A small percentage of colorectal cancers are known to be caused by inherited gene *mutations* (changes in DNA). Recently, scientists have discovered many of these DNA changes, learned how they change growth control of cells, and determined how the changes can be detected in people before colorectal cancers develop.

Changes in a gene called APC are responsible for **familial adenomatous polyposis (FAP)** and Gardner syndrome. This gene is normally responsible for slowing the growth of cells. In patients who have inherited changes in the APC gene, this "brake" on cell growth is turned off and hundreds of polyps develop in the colon. Over time, cancer will nearly always develop in one or more of these polyps because of new gene mutations in the cells of the polyps. We all have these new gene mutations. But they rarely lead to cancer because the cells die instead of continuing to grow as they do when the APC "brake" is turned off.

A defective DNA repair mechanism is responsible for **hereditary nonpolyposis colon cancer (HNPCC)**. Cells must make a new copy of their DNA each time they divide. Occasional errors are made in copying the DNA code. Fortunately, cells have DNA repair enzymes that act like proofreaders or "spell checkers." Mutations in the DNA repair enzyme genes in HNPCC allow DNA errors to go uncorrected. Mutations in at least 4 different genes can lead to errors in repair. These errors will sometimes affect growth-regulating genes. This can lead to the development of cancer.

Tests are available that can detect gene mutations associated with FAP and HNPCC. If you have a family history of colorectal cancer or any of the associated cancers discussed above, you should ask your doctor about genetic counseling and genetic testing. The American Cancer Society recommends discussing genetic testing with a qualified genetic counselor before genetic testing is done.

Most people with colorectal cancer do not have an inherited gene mutation. Instead, the mutations develop spontaneously. Many doctors think the first mutation occurs in the APC gene. This leads to an increased growth of colorectal cells because of the loss of this "brake" molecule. Another mutation then occurs in the gene called K-RAS and causes this gene to become an "accelerator" of cell growth. Many other mutations eventually occur that lead the cells to grow uncontrollably.

Prevention and Detection

Can Colorectal Cancer Be Prevented?

Even though we do not know the exact cause of most colorectal cancer, it is possible to prevent many colorectal cancers.

Screening

One of the most powerful weapons in preventing colorectal cancer is regular colorectal cancer screening or testing. Regular colorectal cancer screening can, in many cases, prevent colorectal cancer altogether. (See the American Cancer Society screening guidelines in the next section, "Can Colorectal Polyps and Cancer Be Found Early?") This is because polyps, or growths, can be detected and removed before they have the chance to turn into cancer. Screening can also result in finding colorectal cancer early, when it is highly curable.

People who have no identified risk factors other than age should begin regular screening at age 50. Those who have a family history or other risk factors for colorectal cancer polyps or cancer need to talk with their doctor about starting screening at a younger age and more frequent intervals.

Diet and exercise

People can lower their risk of developing colorectal cancer by managing the risk factors that they can control, such as diet and physical activity. It is important to eat plenty of fruits, vegetables, and whole grain foods and to limit intake of high-fat foods. Physical activity is another area that people can control. The American Cancer Society recommends at least 30 minutes of physical activity on 5 or more days of the week. If you participate in moderate or vigorous activity for 45 minutes on 5 or more days of the week, you can lower your risk for breast and colorectal cancer even more. If you are overweight, you can ask your doctor about a weight loss plan that will work for you.

Vitamins, calcium, and magnesium

Some studies suggest that taking a daily multivitamin containing folic acid, or folate, can lower colorectal cancer risk. Other studies suggest that increasing calcium intake via supplements or low-fat dairy products will lower risk. Some have suggested that vitamin D, which you can get from sun exposure or in a vitamin pill or in milk, can lower colorectal cancer risk. Indeed the rate of this cancer is lower in the Sunbelt states. Of course, excessive sun exposure can cause skin cancer and is not recommended as a way to lower colorectal cancer risk. Calcium and vitamin D may work together to reduce colorectal cancer risk, as vitamin D aids in the body's absorption of calcium. In addition, a recent study suggested that a diet high in magnesium may also reduce colorectal cancer risk in women.

Nonsteroidal anti-inflammatory drugs

Many studies have found that people who regularly use aspirin and other nonsteroidal anti-inflammatory drugs (NSAIDs), such as ibuprofen (Motrin, Advil) and naproxen (Aleve), have a 20% to 50% lower risk of colorectal cancer and adenomatous polyps. Most of these studies, however, are based on observations of people who took these medications for reasons such as treatment of arthritis or prevention of heart attacks. Two recent studies have provided even stronger evidence regarding aspirin's ability to prevent the growth of polyps. The advantage of these recent studies is that people were randomly selected by the researchers to receive either aspirin or an inactive placebo. One study included people who were previously treated for early stages of colorectal cancer, and the other study included people who previously had polyps removed.

But NSAIDs can cause serious or even life-threatening bleeding from stomach irritation. Currently available information suggests that the risks of serious bleeding outweigh the benefits of these medicines for the general public. For this reason, experts do not recommend NSAIDs as a cancer-prevention strategy for people at average risk of developing colorectal cancer. However, the value of these drugs for people at increased colo-rectal cancer risk is being actively studied. Celecoxib (Celebrex) has been approved by the FDA for reducing polyp formation in people with familial adenomatous polyposis. One advantage of this drug is that it causes less bleeding in the stomach. However, celecoxib is now being investigated for a potential association with increased heart attack and stroke risk. A similar drug, Vioxx, was recently taken off the market because people who took it had an increased number of heart attacks and strokes.

Female hormones

Hormone replacement therapy (HRT) in post-menopausal women may reduce their risk of developing colorectal cancer. But those women on HRT who do develop colorectal cancer may have a fast growing cancer. The reason for this isn't clear, but it means that HRT will probably not lower the chance of dying from this disease.

HRT also lowers the risk of developing osteoporosis, but it may increase the risk of heart disease, blood clots, and breast and uterine cancer. The decision to use HRT should be based on a careful discussion of benefits and risks with your doctor.

Other factors

There are other risk factors that can't be controlled, such as a strong family history of colorectal cancer. But even when people have a history of colorectal cancer in their family, they may be able to prevent the disease. For example, people with a family history of colorectal cancer may benefit from starting screening tests when they are younger and having them done more often than people without this risk factor.

Genetic tests can help determine which members of certain families have inherited a high risk for developing colorectal cancer. Without testing, all members of a family known to have an inherited form of colorectal cancer should be screened frequently. However with testing, family members who are found to not have inherited the gene can be screened with the same frequency as people at average risk.

People with familial adenomatous polyposis (FAP) should start colonoscopy during their teens. Most doctors recommend they have their colon removed when they are in their 20s to prevent cancer from developing.

The lifetime risk of developing colorectal cancer for people with **hereditary nonpolyposis colon cancer (HNPCC)** is about 80% compared with near 100% for those with FAP. Doctors recommend that people with HNPCC start colonoscopy screening during their twenties to remove any polyps and find any cancers at the earliest possible stage. People known to carry the genetic mutation associated with HNPCC may be offered the option of yearly screening with colonoscopy or removal of most of the colon.

Ashkenazi Jews with the I1307K APC mutation have a slightly increased colorectal cancer risk, but do not develop these cancers when they are very young. For these reasons, most doctors recommend that they carefully follow the usual recommendations for colorectal cancer screening, but earlier or more frequent testing is usually not suggested.

Since some colorectal cancers can't be prevented, finding them early is the best way to improve the chance of a cure and reduce the number of deaths caused by this disease.

In addition to the screening recommendations for people at average colorectal cancer risk, the American Cancer Society has additional guidelines for people at moderate and high risk of colorectal cancer. These recommendations are described in the section on "Can Colorectal Cancer Be Found Early?" Ask your doctor how these guidelines might apply to you.

Can Colorectal Polyps and Cancer Be Found Early?

Colorectal Cancer Screening

Screening tests are used to spot a disease early, before you have symptoms or a history of that disease. Screening for colorectal cancer means it can be found at an early curable stage, and it can also be prevented by finding and removing polyps that might eventually become cancerous. There are several tests used to screen for colorectal cancer:

Fecal occult blood test

The **fecal occult blood test (FOBT)** is used to find occult (hidden) blood in feces. Blood vessels at the surface of colorectal polyps or adenomas or cancers are often fragile and easily damaged by the passage of feces. The damaged vessels usually release a small amount of blood into the feces. Only rarely is there enough bleeding to color the stool red. The FOBT detects blood through a chemical reaction. The traditional version of this test cannot tell whether blood is from the colon or from other portions of the digestive tract (i.e., the stomach). Therefore, if this test is positive, a colonoscopy is needed to see if there is a cancer, polyp, or other cause of bleeding such as ulcers, hemorrhoids, diverticulosis (tiny pouches that form at weak spots in the colon wall), or **inflammatory bowel disease (colitis).** Even foods or drugs can affect the test, so some doctors suggest that you should try to avoid the following with this test:

- Nonsteroidal anti-inflammatory drugs (NSAIDS), such as ibuprofen (Advil), naproxen (Aleve), or aspirin (more than 1 adult aspirin per day), for 7 days before testing (they can cause bleeding)
- Vitamin C in excess of 250 mg daily from either supplements or citrus fruits, and juices for 3 days before testing (they can affect the chemicals in the test and make it show <u>negative</u>)
- Red meats for 3 days before testing (components of blood in the meat may cause the test to show <u>positive</u>)
- Raw broccoli, cauliflower, horseradish, parsnips, radishes, turnips and melons for 3 days (peroxidases in these vegetables may cause the test to show <u>positive</u>)

However, research has shown that some people never do the FOBT test or don't give it to their doctor because they worry that something they ate may interfere with the test. For this reason, many doctors tell their patients it isn't essential to follow these restrictions in their diet. The most important thing is to get the test done. People should try to avoid taking aspirin or related drugs for minor aches. But if you take these medications daily for heart problems or other conditions, don't stop them for this test without approval from your doctor.

People having this test will receive a kit with instructions that explain how to take a stool or feces sample at home (usually 3 specimens smeared onto a small square of paper). The kit is then returned to the doctor's office or a medical laboratory for testing. It is not necessary that the kit be returned immediately because the test is still accurate if the smeared feces have dried. A test of a stool sample that your doctor took from a digital rectal exam is not an adequate substitute.

Fecal immunochemical test

A newer kind of stool blood test kit, known as a *fecal immunochemical test* (FIT), detects a specific portion of a human blood protein. This test is done essentially the same way as conventional FOBT, but is more specific and reduces the number of false positive results. Vitamins or foods do not affect the fecal immunochemical test, and some forms require only 2 stool specimens (as opposed to 3 for conventional FOBT), so people may find it easier to use. The fecal immunochemical test has some of the same drawbacks as conventional FOBT, such as an inability to detect a tumor that is not bleeding.

Flexible sigmoidoscopy

A **sigmoidoscope** is a slender, flexible, hollow, lighted tube about the thickness of a finger. It is inserted through the rectum into the lower part of the colon. Not only can your doctor look through this to find any abnormality, the sigmoidoscope can be connected to a video camera and display monitor for a better view. This test may be somewhat uncomfortable, but it should not be painful. Because the sigmoidoscope is only 60 centimeters (around 2 feet) long, the doctor is able to see less than half of the colon with this procedure. Before the sigmoidoscopy, you will need to have a bowel preparation to clean out your lower colon. If an adenomatous polyp or colorectal cancer is found on this examination, you will need to have additional testing such as a colonoscopy to look for polyps of cancer in the rest of the colon.

Colonoscopy

A **colonoscope** is a longer version of a sigmoido-scope. It is inserted through the rectum and allows your doctor to see the lining of your entire colon. The colonoscope is also connected to a video camera and display monitor so the doctor can closely examine the inside of the colon.

If a small polyp is found, your doctor may remove it. Polyps, even those that are not cancerous, can eventually become cancerous. For this reason, they are usually removed. This is done by passing a wire loop through the colonoscope to cut the polyp from the wall of the colon with an electrical current. The polyp can then be sent to a lab to be checked under a microscope to see if it has any areas that have changed into cancer.

If your doctor sees a large polyp or tumor or anything else abnormal, a **biopsy** will be done. In this procedure, a small piece of tissue is taken out through the colonoscope. Examination of the tissue can help determine if it is a cancer, a benign (non-cancerous) growth, or a result of inflammation.

If you have a colonoscopy, you will need to follow a clear-liquid diet and take laxatives the day before the test and an enema that morning to clean your colon so no stool will block the view. Colonoscopy can be uncomfortable. To avoid this, you will be given a sedating medication through a vein to make you feel relaxed and sleepy during the procedure. Colonoscopy may be done in a hospital outpatient department or ambulatory care center and usually takes 15 to 30 minutes, although it may take longer if polyp removal is involved.

Medicare will pay for colonoscopy at specified intervals for all people covered by Medicare who are older than 50.

Barium enema with air contrast

This procedure is also called a **double-contrast barium enema**. Barium sulfate, a chalky substance, is used to partially fill and open up the colon. The barium sulfate is given through a small tube placed in your anus. When the colon is about half-full of barium, you will be turned on the x-ray table so the barium spreads throughout the colon. Then air will be pumped into your colon through the same tube to make it expand. This produces the best pictures of the lining of your colon. You will need to cleanse your bowel the night before with laxatives and have an enema the morning of the exam.

Virtual colonoscopy

This can be thought of as a super x-ray of the colon and rectum. The preparation is the same as for a barium enema x-ray or colonoscopy. No contrast agent is used. Only air is pumped into the colon to distend it. Then a special CT scan called helical CT or spiral CT is done. This is probably more accurate than the barium enema but not quite as good as colonoscopy for finding very small polyps. The potential advantages are believed to be that the test can be done quickly, with no sedation, and at a lower cost than colonoscopy. A disadvantage is that if a polyp or growth is found, a biopsy or polyp removal needs to be done later with a colonoscopy. Virtual colonoscopy is currently not included among the tests recommended by American Cancer Society or other major medical organizations as a screening test for colorectal cancer polyps or for the early detection of colorectal cancer.

American Cancer Society Colorectal Cancer Screening Guidelines

Beginning at age 50, men and women who are at average risk for developing colorectal cancer should have 1 of the 5 screening options below:

1. a **fecal occult blood test (FOBT)*** or **fecal immunochemical test (FIT)** every year, or

2. **flexible sigmoidoscopy** every 5 years, or

3. an FOBT* or FIT every year plus flexible sigmoidoscopy every 5 years, or

   Of these first 3 options, option 3 (the combination of FOBT or FIT every year plus flexible sigmoidoscopy every 5 years) is preferable.

4. **double-contrast barium enema** every 5 years, or

5. **colonoscopy** every 10 years

* For FOBT or FIT, the take-home multiple sample method should be used.

In a **digital rectal examination (DRE),** a doctor examines your rectum with the gloved end of his/her finger. Although a DRE is often included as part of a routine physical exam, it is not recommended as a stand-alone test for colorectal cancer. However, your doctor should do a DRE before inserting the sigmoidoscope or colonoscope. This simple test, which is not painful, can detect masses in the anal canal or lower rectum. By itself, however, it is not a very sensitive test for detecting colorectal cancer due to its limited reach.

American Cancer Society Guidelines on Screening and Surveillance for the Early Detection of Colorectal Adenomas and Cancer – Women and Men at Increased Risk or at High Risk

Risk Category	Age to Begin	Recommendation	Comment
INCREASED RISK			
People with a single, small (< 1 cm) adenoma	3-6 years after the initial polypectomy	Colonoscopy[1]	If the exam is normal, the patient can thereafter be screened as per average risk guidelines.
People with a large (1 cm +) adenoma, multiple adenomas, or adenomas with high-grade dysplasia or villous change	Within 3 years after the initial polypectomy	Colonoscopy[1]	If normal, repeat examination in 3 years; If normal then, the patient can thereafter be screened as per average risk . guidelines
Personal history of curative-intent resection of colorectal cancer	Within 1 year after cancer resection	Colonoscopy[1]	If normal, repeat examination in 3 years; If normal then, repeat examination every 5 years.
Either colorectal cancer or adeno-matous polyps, in any first-degree relative before age 60, or in two or more first-degree relatives at any age (if not a hereditary syndrome)	Age 40, or 10 years before the youngest case in the immediate family, whichever is earlier	Colonoscopy[1]	Every 5-10 years. Colorectal cancer in relatives more distant than first-degree does not increase risk substantially above the average risk group.

HIGH RISK

Family history of familial adenomatous polyposis (FAP)	Puberty	Early surveillance with endoscopy, and counseling to consider genetic testing	If the genetic test is positive, colectomy is indicated. These patients are best referred to a center with experience in the management of FAP.
Family history of hereditary non-polyposis colon cancer (HNPCC)	Age 21	Colonoscopy and counseling to consider genetic testing	If the genetic test is positive or if the patient has not had genetic testing, every 1-2 years until age 40, then annually. These patients are best referred to a center with experience in the management of HNPCC.
Inflammatory bowel disease: -Chronic ulcerative colitis -Crohn's disease	Cancer risk begins to be significant 8 years after the onset of pancolitis, or 12-15 years after the onset of left-sided colitis	Colonoscopy with biopsies for dysplasia every 1-2 years	These patients are best referred to a center with experience in the surveillance and management of inflammatory bowel disease.

[1] *If colonoscopy is unavailable, not feasible, or not desired by the patient, double-contrast barium enema (DCBE) alone, or the combination of flexible sigmoidoscopy and DCBE are acceptable alternatives. Adding flexible sigmoidoscopy to DCBE may provide a more comprehensive diagnostic evaluation than DCBE alone in finding significant lesions. A supplementary DCBE may be needed if a colonoscopic exam fails to reach the cecum, and a supplementary colonoscopy may be needed if a DCBE identifies a possible lesion, or does not adequately visualize the entire colon and rectum.*

Colonoscopy should be done if the FOBT or FIT shows blood in the stool, if sigmoidoscopy results show a polyp, or if double-contrast barium enema studies find anything abnormal. If possible, polyps should be removed during the colonoscopy.

You should begin colorectal cancer screening earlier and/or undergo screening more often if you have any of the following colorectal cancer risk factors:

- a strong family history of colorectal cancer or polyps (cancer or polyps in a first-degree relative [parent, sibling, or child] younger than 60, or in 2 first-degree relatives of any age)
- a known family history of hereditary colorectal cancer syndromes (familial adenomatous polyposis and hereditary nonpolyposis colon cancer)
- a personal history of colorectal cancer or adenomatous polyps
- a personal history of chronic inflammatory bowel disease

The table on the previous page suggests screening guidelines for those with an *increased or high risk* of colorectal cancer, based on specific risk factors. Some people may have more than 1 risk factor. Please refer to this table and discuss these recommendations with your doctor. Based on your individual situation and any risk factors you may have, your doctor can suggest which screening option is best for you as well as any modifications in the schedule based on your individual risk.

Medicare Coverage for Colorectal Screening

What Colorectal Cancer Screening Is Covered by Medicare?

- **Fecal occult blood test** (FOBT) or **fecal immunochemical test** (FIT) yearly for all Medicare beneficiaries 50 years and older
- **Flexible sigmoidoscopy** (flex-sig) every 4 years for beneficiaries 50 years and older who are at average risk
- **Colonoscopy** every 2 years for all beneficiaries at high risk
- **Colonoscopy** once every 10 years for beneficiaries age 50 and older who are at average risk
- **Double contrast barium enema** (**DCBE**) as an alternative if a physician determines that its screening value is equal to or better than flexible sigmoidoscopy or colonoscopy

What Would a Medicare Beneficiary Expect to Pay for a Colorectal Cancer Screening Test?

- **FOBT/FIT:** People age 50 years or older with Medicare pay no coinsurance and no Part B deductible.
- **Flexible sigmoidoscopy:** Patient pays 20% of Medicare-approved amount after the yearly Part B deductible.
- **Colonoscopy:** Patient pays 20% of Medicare-approved amount after the yearly Part B deductible.

- **DCBE:** When substituted for flexible sigmoidoscopy or colonoscopy, patient pays 20% of Medicare-approved amount after the yearly Part B deductible.

Diagnosis and Staging

How Is Colorectal Cancer Diagnosed?

Most people with early colon cancer have no symptoms of the disease. Symptoms usually appear only with more advanced disease. You will need to undergo a diagnostic workup if your doctor finds something suspicious during a screening examination or if you have symptoms of colorectal cancer.

If you have any such symptoms, please see your doctor immediately. He or she will need to take a complete medical history and perform a physical exam to determine the cause of your symptoms. Additional tests may be done to find out if you have colorectal cancer, or a different condition that may have some of the same symptoms.

Signs and Symptoms of Colorectal Cancer

If you have any of the following you should check with your doctor for prompt diagnosis and treatment:

- a change in bowel habits such as diarrhea, constipation, or narrowing of the stool that lasts for more than a few days
- a feeling that you need to have a bowel movement that is not relieved by doing so

- rectal bleeding or blood in the stool (often, though, the stool will look normal)
- cramping or steady abdominal (stomach area) pain
- weakness and fatigue

Other conditions, such as infections, hemorrhoids, and inflammatory bowel disease, can also cause these symptoms. But only a doctor can determine their cause. It is important to talk to your doctor since finding colorectal cancer early makes successful treatment more likely. It is also possible to have colon cancer and not have any symptoms. If the doctor suspects colon cancer, you may need to have more tests done. Remember that most people with colorectal cancer have normal-looking stools.

Whether you are undergoing diagnosis because of the results of a screening exam or because you have symptoms, your doctor may perform the following:

Medical history and physical exam

When your doctor "takes a history," he or she will ask you a series of questions about your symptoms and risk factors, including your family history. Your doctor will carefully examine your abdomen to feel for masses or enlarged organs, and also examine the rest of your body. Your doctor may also perform a digital rectal examination (DRE).

FOBT, sigmoidoscopy, barium enema, double-contrast barium enema, colonoscopy

Your doctor may recommend one or more of these tests to further investigate a suspicious finding or determine the cause of your symptoms.

Blood tests

Your doctor may also order a blood count. This will determine whether you are anemic. Many people with colorectal cancer become anemic because of prolonged bleeding from the tumor. You may also have a blood test of your liver function, because colorectal cancer can spread to the liver and cause abnormalities.

In addition, colorectal cancer produces substances such as carcinoembryonic antigen (CEA) and CA 19-9 that are released into the bloodstream. Blood tests for these "tumor markers" are used most often with other tests for follow-up of patients who already have been treated for colorectal cancer. They may provide an early warning of a cancer that has returned.

These tumor markers are not used to find cancer in people who have never had a cancer and appear to be healthy. Tumor marker levels can be normal in a person who has cancer and can be abnormal for reasons other than cancer. For example, higher levels may also be present in the blood of some people with ulcerative colitis, non-cancerous tumors of the intestines, or some types of liver disease or chronic lung disease. Smoking can also raise CEA levels.

Biopsy

Usually, if a suspected colorectal cancer is found by any test, it is biopsied during colonoscopy. In a biopsy, the doctor removes a small piece of tissue. This is sent to the pathology laboratory where a pathologist, a doctor especially trained to diagnose cancer and other diseases in tissue samples, examines the tissue under a microscope.

Imaging Tests

Ultrasound

Ultrasound involves the use of sound waves and their echoes to produce a picture of internal organs or masses. A small microphone-like instrument called a *transducer* emits sound waves. These high-frequency sound waves are transmitted into the area of the body being studied and echoed back. The sound wave echoes are picked up by the transducer and converted by a computer into an image that is displayed on a computer screen. Abdominal ultrasound can look for tumors in your liver, gallbladder, pancreas, or even inside your abdomen. It can't look for tumors of the colon.

This is a very easy procedure. It uses no radiation, which is why it is frequently used to look at developing fetuses. When you undergo an ultrasound examination, you simply lie on a table and a technician moves the transducer over the skin overlying the part of your body being examined. Usually, the skin is first lubricated with oil.

Two special types of ultrasound examinations can be used to evaluate people with colon and rectal cancer. *Endorectal ultrasound* uses a special transducer that can be inserted directly into the rectum. This test is used to see how far through the wall a rectal cancer may have penetrated and whether it has spread to nearby organs or tissues such as lymph nodes. *Intraoperative ultrasound* is done after the surgeon has opened the abdominal cavity. The transducer can be placed against the surface of the liver, making this test very useful in detecting metastases of colorectal cancer to the liver.

Computed tomography (CT)

The CT scan is an x-ray procedure that produces detailed cross-sectional images of your body. Instead of taking one picture, as does a conventional x-ray, a CT scanner takes many pictures as it rotates around you. A computer then combines these pictures into an image of a slice of your body. The machine will take pictures of multiple slices of the part of your body that is being studied. This test can help tell if your colon cancer has spread into your liver or other organs. Often after the first set of pictures is taken you will receive an intra-venous injection of a dye (a *contrast agent*) that helps outline structures in your body. A second set of pictures is then taken. You may be asked to drink 1 to 2 pints of a solution of contrast material. This helps outline the intestine so that it is not mistaken for tumors.

A special kind of CT, the *spiral CT*, uses a special scanner that can provide greater detail and is sometimes useful in finding metastases from colorectal cancer. For spiral CT with portography (looking at the portal vein —the large vein leading into the liver from the intes-tine), contrast material is injected into veins that lead to the liver, to help find metastases from colorectal cancer to that organ.

CT scans can also be used to precisely guide a biopsy needle into a suspected metastasis. For this procedure, called a *CT-guided needle biopsy*, the patient remains on the CT scanning table, while a radiologist advances a biopsy needle toward the location of the mass. CT scans are repeated until the doctors are confident that the needle is within the mass. A fine needle biopsy sample (tiny fragment of tissue) or a core needle biopsy sample (a thin cylinder of tissue about ½ inch long and less than ⅛ inch in diameter) is removed and examined under a microscope.

CT scans are more tedious than regular x-rays because they take longer and you need to lie still on a table while they are being done. But they are getting faster and your stay might be pleasantly short. Also, you might feel a bit confined by the ring you lie within when the pictures are being taken.

You will need to put up with the intravenous (IV) line through which the contrast dye is injected. The injection can also cause some flushing. Some people are allergic and get hives or, rarely, more serious reactions like trouble breathing and low blood pressure. Please be sure to tell the doctor if you have ever had a reaction to any contrast material used for x-rays.

A new experimental application of the CT is to perform a "virtual colonoscopy." After cleansing the stool from the colon and filling the colon with air, a computer-assisted reconstruction of the colon from CT images is possible. It requires the same preparation as for a colonoscopy. Also, the colon is inflated with air so that it can be viewed more clearly; this stretches the colon and can cause some discomfort. If abnormalities are detected, a follow-up colonoscopy will be required to take tissue samples of the abnormal areas.

Magnetic resonance imaging (MRI)

MRI scans involve the use of radio waves and strong magnets instead of x-rays. The energy from the radio waves is absorbed and then released in a pattern formed by the type of tissue and by certain diseases. A computer translates the pattern of radio waves given off by the tissues into a detailed image of parts of the body. Not only does this produce cross-sectional slices of the body like a CT scanner, it can also produce slices that are parallel with the length of your body. A contrast material might be injected just as with CT scans, but is used less often.

MRI scans are particularly helpful in examining the brain and spinal cord. MRI scans are a little more uncomfortable than CT scans. First, they take longer— often up to an hour. Also, you often have to be placed inside a tube, which is confining and can upset people with a fear of enclosed spaces. The machine also makes a thumping noise, but some places will provide headphones with music to block this out.

Chest x-ray

This test may be done to determine whether colorectal cancer has spread to the lungs.

Positron emission tomography (PET)

PET scans involve the use of glucose (a form of sugar) that contains a radioactive atom. A small amount of the radioactive material is injected into your arm. Then you are put into the PET machine where a special camera can detect the radioactivity. Because of their high rate of metabolism, cancer cells absorb large amounts of the radioactive sugar. PET is useful when your doctor thinks the cancer has spread, but doesn't know to where. PET scans can be used instead of several different x-rays because it scans your whole body and may find spread of the cancer where CT scans haven't. PET scans have become more accurate because newer devices combine the PET scan with a CT scan. This test is known as integrated PET/CT.

Angiography

For this test, doctors insert a very thin tube into a blood vessel that goes to the area to be studied. Contrast dye is injected rapidly and a series of x-ray images is then taken. This can show surgeons the location of blood vessels next to a liver metastasis from colorectal cancer, so that they can remove the metastasis without causing a lot of bleeding.

How Is Colorectal Cancer Staged?

Staging is a process that tells the doctor how widespread your cancer may be at the time of diagnosis. It will show whether the cancer has spread and how far. The treatment and outlook for colorectal cancer depends, to a large extent, on its stage. For early cancer, surgery may be all that is needed. For more advanced cancer, other treatments, such as chemotherapy or radiation therapy, may be required. Please be sure to ask your doctor to explain the stage of your cancer so that you can make the best choice about your treatment.

More than one system is used for staging colorectal cancer. These include the Dukes, Astler-Coller, and AJCC/TNM systems. This section concentrates on American Joint Committee on Cancer (AJCC) system (also called the TNM system), which describes stages using Roman numerals I through IV. Both the Dukes system and the Astler-Coller system use A through C; the Astler-Coller system adds stage D and has more subdivisions.

All 3 systems describe the spread of the cancer in relation to the layers of the wall of the colon or rectum, organs next to the colon and rectum, and other organs farther away. Because for most patients this stage is unknown until after surgery, most doctors wait till then to decide on the cancer's stage. The stages described below are called **pathologic stages**. The pathologic stage is determined by the findings of the pathologist from looking at the cancer and other actual tissue that has been removed.

The AJCC / TNM System describes the extent of the primary **T**umor (T), the absence or presence of metastasis to nearby lymph **N**odes (N), and the absence or presence of distant **M**etastasis (M).

T Categories for Colorectal Cancer

T categories of colorectal cancer describe the extent of spread through the layers that form the wall of the colon and rectum. These layers, from the inner to the outer, include the lining (**mucosa**), the fibrous tissue beneath this muscle layer (*submucosa*), a thick layer of muscle that contracts to force the contents of the intestines along (*muscularis propria*), and the thin outermost layers of connective tissue (*subserosa and serosa*) that cover most of the colon but not the rectum.

- **Tx:** No description of the tumor's extent is possible because of incomplete information.
- **Tis:** The cancer is in the earliest stage. It has not grown beyond the mucosa (inner layer) of the colon or rectum. This stage is also known as carcinoma in situ or intramucosal carcinoma.
- **T1:** The cancer has grown through the mucosa and extends into the submucosa.
- **T2:** The cancer has grown through the submucosa and extends into the muscularis propria.

- **T3:** The cancer has grown completely through the muscularis propria into the subserosa but not to any neighboring organs or tissues.
- **T4:** The cancer has spread completely through the wall of the colon or rectum into nearby tissues or organs.

N Categories for Colorectal Cancer

N categories indicate whether or not the cancer has spread to nearby lymph nodes and, if so, how many lymph nodes are involved.

- **Nx:** No description of lymph node involvement is possible because of incomplete information.
- **N0:** No lymph node involvement is found.
- **N1:** Cancer cells found in 1 to 3 nearby lymph nodes.
- **N2:** Cancer cells found in 4 or more nearby lymph nodes.

M Categories for Colorectal Cancer

M categories indicate whether or not the cancer has spread to distant organs, such as the liver, lungs, or distant lymph nodes.

- **Mx:** No description of distant spread is possible because of incomplete information.
- **M0:** No distant spread is seen.
- **M1:** Distant spread is present.

Stage Grouping

Once a person's T, N, and M categories have been determined, usually after surgery, this information is combined in a process called *stage grouping* to determine the stage, expressed in Roman numerals from stage I (the least advanced stage) to stage IV (the most advanced stage). The following guide illustrates how TNM categories are grouped together into stages:

- **Stage 0: Tis, N0, M0:** The cancer is in the earliest stage. It has not grown beyond the inner layer (mucosa) of the colon or rectum. This stage is also known as carcinoma in situ or intramucosal carcinoma.

- **Stage I: T1, N0, M0, or T2, N0, M0:** The cancer has grown through the mucosa into the submucosa or it may also have grown into the muscularis propria, but it has not spread into nearby lymph nodes or distant sites.

- **Stage IIA: T3, N0, M0:** The cancer has grown through the wall of the colon or rectum into the outermost layers. It has not yet spread to the nearby lymph nodes or distant sites.

- **Stage IIB: T4, N0, M0:** The cancer has grown through the wall of the colon or rectum into other nearby tissues or organs. It has not yet spread to the nearby lymph nodes or distant sites.

- **Stage IIIA: T1-2, N1, M0:** The cancer has grown through the mucosa into the submucosa or it may also have grown into the muscularis propria, and it has spread to 1-3 nearby lymph nodes but not distant sites.

- **Stage IIIB: T3-4, N1, M0:** The cancer has grown through the wall of the colon or rectum or into other nearby tissues or organs and has spread to 1-3 nearby lymph nodes but not distant sites.

- **Stage IIIC: Any T, N2, M0:** The cancer can be any T but has spread to 4 or more nearby lymph nodes but not distant sites.
- **Stage IV: Any T, Any N, M1:** The cancer can be any T, any N, but has spread to distant sites such as the liver, lung, peritoneum (the membrane lining the abdominal cavity), or ovary.

Comparison of AJCC, Dukes, and Astler-Coller Stages

If your stage is reported in letters rather than numbers, this table can be used to find the matching AJCC/TNM stage. As you can see, the Dukes and Astler-Coller staging systems often combine different AJCC stage groupings and are not as precise.

AJCC/TNM	Dukes	Astler-Coller
0		
I	A	A, B1
IIA	B	B2
IIB	B	B3
IIIA	C	C1,
IIIB	C	C2, C3
IIIC	C	C1, C2, C3
IV	D	

If you have any questions about your stage, please ask your doctor to explain the extent of your disease.

*Five-year relative survival by AJCC stage**

These numbers reflect the percent of people who are alive 5 years or more after being diagnosed with colon cancer, depending on what stage they were in when they were diagnosed. See below for definition of 5-year relative survival. The survival for rectal cancer, stage for stage, is about the same**.

Stage I	93%
Stage IIA	85%
Stage IIB	72%
Stage IIIA	83%
Stage IIIB	64%
Stage IIIC	44%
Stage IV	8%

*JNCI 2004;96:1420
**NCDB Commission on Cancer

The 5-year survival rate refers to the percentage of patients who live at least 5 years after their cancer is diagnosed. Many of these patients live much longer than 5 years after diagnosis. The 5-year rate is used to produce a standard way of discussing prognosis. **Five-year relative survival rates** don't include patients dying of other diseases. Five-year relative survival rates are considered to be a more accurate way to describe the prognosis for patients with a particular type and stage of cancer. Of course, 5-year rates are based on patients diagnosed and initially treated more than 5 years ago. They may no longer be accurate because improvements in treatment may result in a better outlook for recently diagnosed patients.

Five-year relative survival for patients with rectal cancer by AJCC stage treated 1990-1999*. (These stages are slightly different from those above. They come from the third edition, 1988):

*The Oncologist 2003;8:541 (See complete citation in the References section, page 97.)

Stage I	92%
Stage II	73%
Stage III	56%
Stage IV	8%

In an update that used patients from 1991-1993 that were stage III and divided them according to the staging above (6th Edition) into stage IIIa, IIIb, IIIc these results were obtained for relative 5-year survival:

Stage IIIA	67%
Stage IIIB	44%
Stage IIIC	30%

Another factor that contributes to the outlook for survival is the grade of the cancer. Grade is a description of how closely the cancer resembles normal colorectal tissue. Low grade means the tissue closely resembles normal tissue and high grade means the tissue appears most unlike normal tissue. Most of the time, high-grade cancers are associated with a poorer outcome than low-grade cancers. Doctors sometimes use this distinction to decide whether a patient should get extra treatment with chemotherapy after surgery.

Treatments

How Is Colorectal Cancer Treated?

The following information is a summary of the types of treatments available to people with colorectal cancer. The usual treatments for colorectal cancers at each stage are then discussed.

The 3 main types of treatment for colon cancer and rectal cancer are surgery, radiation therapy, and chemotherapy. Newer, targeted therapies called monoclonal antibodies are now beginning to be used as well. Depending on the stage of the cancer, 2 or more of these types of treatment may be combined at the same time or used one after another.

After the cancer has been found and staged, your doctor will recommend one or more treatment options. It is important to take time and think about all of the choices. You may want to ask for a second opinion. This can provide more information and help you feel more confident about the treatment plan you choose. It is also important to know that your chances for having the best possible outcome are highest in the hands of a medical team that is experienced in treating colorectal cancer.

Surgery

Colon surgery

Surgery is the main treatment for colon cancer. The most commonly performed operation is called a **segmental resection**. To prepare for this surgery you will be given a bowel prep which may consist of laxatives and enemas. Just before the surgery you will be given general anesthesia, which puts you into a deep sleep. During the surgery, your surgeon will make an incision in your abdomen. Then he or she will remove the cancer and a length of normal colon on either side of your cancer, as well as the nearby lymph nodes. Usually, about one-fourth to one-third of your colon is removed, but more or less tissue may be removed depending on the exact size and location of your cancer. The remaining sections of your colon are then reattached. When you wake up you will have some pain and will need to be given painkillers, usually morphine, for 2 or 3 days.

For the first couple of days, you will be given intravenous fluids and not be able to eat. But a colon resection rarely causes any major problems with digestive functions and you should be able to eat in a few days. If the tumor is large and has blocked your colon, or it has punched a hole in your colon so wastes have leaked out, a temporary **colostomy** may be needed. A colostomy is made when the end of the colon is brought through an opening in the abdomen to the outside for the purpose of getting rid of body wastes. A pouch is then used to hold that waste. Rarely, if a tumor can't be removed, a permanent colostomy is needed.

It is possible to remove some very early colon cancers (stage 0 and some stage I tumors), or cancerous polyps, by surgery through a colonoscope. When this is done, the surgeon does not have to cut into the abdomen. This is called a **polypectomy**. The cancer is cut out across the base of the polyp's *stalk*, the area that resembles the stem of a mushroom. Local excision removes superficial cancers and a small amount of nearby tissue.

It is sometimes possible to remove segments of the colon and nearby lymph nodes through a laparoscope. This is sometimes called "laparoscopic" or "keyhole" surgery. Using a *canula* (a narrow tube-like instrument), the surgeon enters the abdomen. A **laparoscope** (a tiny telescope connected to a video camera) is inserted through the canula, giving the surgeon a magnified view of the internal organs, which is displayed on a television monitor. Several other canulas are inserted to allow the surgeon to work inside and remove part of the colon. These incisions are usually small and heal quickly. Although using laparoscopic surgery to remove colon cancers was once considered experimental, this is no longer true. A recent study has shown that laparoscopic surgery is as likely to be curative as the standard approach and patients recover faster and feel better than they do after conventional colon surgery.

Rectal surgery

Surgery is usually the main treatment for rectal cancer, although radiation and chemotherapy may also be used in addition to surgery. Several surgical methods are used for removing or destroying rectal cancers.

Polypectomy and local excision can be used to remove superficial cancers or polyps. *Local transanal*

resection involves cutting through all layers of the rectum to remove invasive cancers as well as some surrounding normal rectal tissue. Polypectomy, local excision, and local transanal resection are done with instruments inserted through the anus, without making a surgical opening in the skin of the abdomen. This procedure can be used to remove some stage I rectal cancers that are relatively small and not too far from the anus.

Some stage I rectal cancers and most stage II or III rectal cancers are removed by either *low anterior resection* or *abdominoperineal* (AP) *resection.* Low anterior resection is used for cancers in the upper two thirds of your rectum, close to where it connects with the colon. In this procedure the tumor can be removed without affecting the anus. After low anterior resection, your colon will be attached to the anus and your waste will be eliminated in the usual way.

A low anterior resection is like most abdominal operations. You will take laxatives and enemas before surgery. Just before surgery you will be given general anesthesia, which puts you into a deep sleep. The surgeon makes the incision only in the abdomen. Then the surgeon removes the cancer along with a margin of normal tissue on either side of the cancer. In addition, the surgeon will also remove lymph nodes and a large amount of fatty and fibrous tissue around the rectum. Then the colon can be reattached to the rectum that is remaining so that a permanent colostomy is not necessary. Sometimes, when special techniques are necessary to prevent a permanent colostomy, you may need to have a temporary colostomy opening for about 8 weeks while the surgical site heals. A second operation is then performed to close the temporary colostomy opening.

If the cancer is in the distal third of the rectum (the part nearest to the anus) and especially if it is growing into the sphincter muscle (the muscle that keeps the anus closed and prevents stool leakage), the anus and sphincter muscle may also need to be removed. Then an operation called an *abdominoperineal resection* is necessary. Here, not only does the surgeon make an incision in the abdomen, he or she must also make an incision in the perineal area around the anus. This incision allows the surgeon to remove the anus and the tissues surrounding it including the sphincter muscle. Having this procedure also means you will need a permanent colostomy to eliminate your stool.

The usual hospital stay for either of these procedures is 4 to 7 days depending on your overall health. Recovery time at home may be 3 to 6 weeks. If you have had a colostomy, you will need help in learning how to manage it. Specially trained *ostomy nurses* or **enterostomal therapists** can do this. They will usually see you in the hospital before your operation to mark a site for the colostomy opening, and later can come to your house or an outpatient setting to provide you with more training.

If the rectal cancer is growing into nearby organs, a *pelvic exenteration* may be recommended. This is a very extensive operation. Not only will the surgeon remove your rectum, but also nearby organs such as the bladder, prostate, or uterus when the cancer has spread to these organs. You will need a colostomy after pelvic exenteration. If your bladder is removed, you will also need a *urostomy* (opening where urine exits the front of the abdomen and is held in a portable pouch).

Side effects of surgery

Side effects include bleeding from the surgery, blood clots in the legs, and damage to nearby organs during the operation. Rarely, the connections between the ends of the intestine may not hold together completely and leak. If an infection occurs, it is possible that the incision might open up, causing a gaping wound. Later, after the surgery, you might develop what are called adhesions that could cause the bowel to become blocked.

Sexual impact of colorectal surgery

If you are a man, an abdominal perineal resection can cause you to have "dry" orgasms by damaging the nerves that control ejaculation. Sometimes the surgery only causes retrograde ejaculation, which means the semen goes backward into your bladder. The difference between no emission at all and retrograde ejaculation becomes important if you want to father a child. Retrograde ejaculation is less serious, because infertility specialists can recover sperm cells from your urine and these cells can be used to make a woman pregnant. If sperm cells cannot be recovered from your semen or urine, infertility specialists may be able to retrieve them directly from your testicle by minor surgery, and then use them for in vitro fertilization to produce a pregnancy. In some situations, AP resection may stop your erections or ability to reach orgasm. In other cases your pleasure at orgasm may become less intense. Normal aging may cause some of these changes, but they may be made worse by the surgery.

If you are a woman having a colostomy, you should not normally expect any loss of sexual function.

Surgical treatment of colorectal cancer metastases

Sometimes, treatment of cancer that has spread to other organs, or metastasized, can help you to live longer—or even to be cured. If only a small number of metastases are present in the liver, lungs, or ovaries, they may be removed by surgery. If only a few liver metastases are present, completely removing them along with the colorectal tumor may even cure you. Liver metastases may also be destroyed by freezing them (*cryosurgery*), by heating them with microwaves, by injecting material into large blood vessels feeding the tumor to block blood flow (*embolization*), or by injecting concentrated alcohol into the tumor. These methods do not require a surgical operation. The freezing probe, microwave probe, or needle is inserted through the skin and guided to the tumor by CT scans or ultrasound images. However, these methods are not curative.

Radiation Therapy

Radiation therapy uses high-energy rays that destroy cancer cells. After surgery for rectal cancer, radiation can kill small deposits of cancer that may not be seen during surgery. If a rectal cancer's size and/or position make surgery difficult, radiation may be used before surgery to shrink the tumor. Radiation also may be used to ease (*palliate*) symptoms if you have advanced cancer causing intestinal blockage, bleeding, or pain. Chemotherapy can make radiation therapy more effective against some colon and rectal cancers, and these 2 treatments are often used together.

The main use for radiation therapy in people with colon cancer is when the cancer has attached to an internal organ or the lining of the abdomen. When this occurs, the surgeon cannot be certain that all the cancer has been removed, and radiation therapy is used to kill the cancer cells remaining after surgery. For rectal cancer, radiation therapy is usually given to prevent the cancer from coming back in the pelvis where the tumor started. It may be given either before or after surgery, but recently doctors have begun to favor preoperative treatment, along with chemotherapy. Radiation therapy is given to treat local recurrences in rectal cancers that are causing symptoms such as pain. Radiation therapy is seldom used to treat metastatic colon cancer because of side effects and relative resistance when given at the lower tolerated doses.

External-beam radiation therapy focuses radiation on the cancer from a machine outside the body called a *linear accelerator*. This is the type of radiation therapy most often recommended for people with colon cancer. Treatments are given 5 days a week for several weeks. Each treatment lasts only a few minutes and is similar to having a diagnostic x-ray test. As with a diagnostic x-ray, the radiation passes through the skin and other tissues before it reaches the tumor. The actual radiation exposure is very quick, and most of the time is spent precisely positioning the patient so that the radiation is aimed accurately at the cancer.

Endocavitary radiation therapy, like external-beam radiation therapy, is delivered from a radiation source outside the body. It is a hand-held device that is placed into the anus. The device delivers high-intensity radiation over a few minutes. This is repeated about 3 more times at about 2-week intervals for the full dose. The advantage is that the radiation is aimed through the anus and reaches the rectum without passing through the skin and other tissues of the abdomen. This can allow some patients, particularly elderly persons, to avoid radical surgery and colostomy. It is used only for small tumors. Sometimes external beam therapy is also given.

Brachytherapy (internal radiation therapy) uses small pellets of radioactive material placed next to or directly into the cancer. Internal radiation is sometimes used in treating people with rectal cancer, particularly sick or elderly people who would not be able to tolerate curative surgery. This is generally a one-time only procedure and doesn't require daily visits for several weeks.

Side effects of radiation therapy

Side effects of radiation therapy for colon and rectal cancer include mild skin irritation, nausea, diarrhea, rectal irritation, bladder irritation, fatigue, or sexual problems (impotence in men and vaginal irritation in women). Most of these will lessen after treatments are completed. The sexual problems and rectal and bladder irritation can persist. Some degree of rectal and/or bladder irritation may be a permanent side effect. This can lead to diarrhea, bleeding, and frequent urination. If you have these or other side effects, talk to your doctor. There may be ways to lessen many of them.

Chemotherapy

Use of chemotherapy after surgery can increase the survival rate for patients with some stages of colon cancer and rectal cancer. This is called **adjuvant** (additional) chemotherapy. It is given when there is no evidence of cancer but there is a chance that it might come back. Chemotherapy can also help shrink tumors and relieve symptoms of advanced cancer. This is called **palliative** chemotherapy.

Systemic chemotherapy uses anticancer drugs that are injected into a vein or given by mouth. These drugs enter the bloodstream and reach all areas of the body. This treatment is useful for cancers that have metastasized (spread) beyond the organ they started in. In *regional chemotherapy*, drugs are injected directly into an artery leading to a part of the body containing a tumor. This approach concentrates the dose of chemotherapy reaching the cancer cells. It reduces side effects by limiting the amount reaching the rest of the body. *Hepatic artery infusion* is an example of regional chemotherapy sometimes used for colon cancer that has spread to the liver.

Fluorouracil (5-FU) is the drug most often used to treat colon cancer. In adjuvant therapy, it is often given together with another drug, *leucovorin*, which increases its effectiveness. In the past, 5-FU was usually injected slowly into a vein over about 5 minutes and then followed by the leucovorin. These injections were given daily for 5 days, followed by 3 weeks off chemotherapy or weekly for 6 weeks, followed by 2 weeks off treatment.

Recently it has been found that a different way of giving these drugs may be better. In this regimen, called the de Gramont regimen, the 5-FU is given continuously over 2 days as well as by rapid injection on the first day. The leucovorin is given on the first and second day over 2 hours. The de Gramont regimen is given every other week.

In all of these schedules, alternating periods of treatment and recovery are repeated over a period of 6 months to 1 year. In some regimens the 5-FU is given continuously and patients wear a small battery-operated pump that continuously infuses 5-FU into an intravenous catheter. Leucovorin and 5-FU are also used for palliative treatment (to control the growth of the cancer or relieve symptoms). Generally, 5-FU/leucovorin is given for 6 months.

Capecitabine (Xeloda) is an oral chemotherapy drug that is changed to 5-FU once it gets to the tumor site. This drug can be used instead of intravenous 5-FU and acts as if the 5-FU were being given continuously. The side effects of treatment with this drug are nausea, diarrhea, and a syndrome of hand and foot redness that is sometimes accompanied by skin peeling.

Irinotecan (Camptosar) is often used to help control colorectal cancer. It formerly was used in patients no longer responding to palliative 5-FU therapy. But it has been found that irinotecan combined with 5-FU and leucovorin is more effective than 5-FU and leucovorin alone as the first treatment in people with metastatic colorectal cancer, so it is now often used as the first treatment in this situation. This combination may also be more effective as an adjuvant therapy after surgery. Clinical trials have begun to study whether irinotecan would be effective in preventing recurrence.

Although adding irinotecan to the standard chemotherapy combination of 5-FU and leucovorin makes the treatment more effective, it may also make your side effects (such as diarrhea, nausea, and low white blood cell counts) more severe. Irinotecan can cause severe diarrhea, so you must tell your doctor right away if you develop diarrhea. Your doctors may not recommend irinotecan if you are elderly or have other serious health problems. If these severe side effects are uncontrolled, they may lead to death.

These side effects are not as much a problem in patients who do well with the first treatment. If you are already on this combination and have not had any major problems, you are probably safe.

Oxaliplatin (Eloxatin) is another drug recently approved by the FDA for use in colorectal cancer. Oxaliplatin is very effective when combined with 5-FU and leucovorin (LV). The major side effect of oxaliplatin is that it causes numbness and tingling—and extreme sensitivity to temperature—in various parts of the body, mostly arms and legs. This can last for months but almost always goes away in most patients. But about 12% of patients who receive this drug as adjuvant therapy will have long-lasting nerve damage. Just recently, a new drug was found to reduce the numbness and tingling associated with oxaliplatin. If you are taking oxaliplatin, talk with your doctor about side effects beforehand, and to let him or her know as soon as you develop numbness and tingling, or other side effects.

Patients with more advanced cancers, which includes some with stage II and all with stage III have a higher chance that the cancer will return, often at a distant site.

Many clinical trials have tested different combinations of drugs to prevent this recurrence. The most effective adjuvant treatment seems to be a chemotherapy combination called FOLFOX (**Fol**inic acid, 5-**FU**, **Ox**aliplatin). This is a combination of 5-FU and leucovorin (also called folinic acid) given by the de Gramont method along with oxaliplatin. Another regimen gives the 5-FU and leucovorin weekly by rapid intravenous infusion along with the oxaliplatin. Although this may be as effective as FOLFOX 4, it appears to have more side effects, mainly causing severe diarrhea. Other regimens that may be used are combinations of 5-FU and leucovorin.

Side effects of chemotherapy

Chemotherapy drugs kill cancer cells but also damage some normal cells. Your doctor and other health providers can help to avoid or minimize side effects, which will depend on the type of drugs, the amount taken, and the length of your treatment. You might temporarily experience nausea and vomiting, loss of appetite, loss of hair, hand and foot swelling and rashes, and mouth sores. Diarrhea can be troubling, especially if you are receiving irinotecan (Camptosar), but it can also occur with 5-FU/leucovorin treatment. Nerve damage from oxaliplatin can also be troubling but eventually disappears.

Because chemotherapy can damage the blood-producing cells of the bone marrow, you may develop low blood cell counts. This can result in an increased chance of infection (due to a shortage of white blood cells), bleeding or bruising after minor cuts or injuries (due to a shortage of blood platelets), and fatigue (due to low red blood cell counts). Please talk with your doctor if you have any unrelieved side effects.

Most side effects disappear once treatment is stopped. Your hair will grow back after treatment ends, though it may look different. There are remedies for many of the temporary side effects of chemotherapy— for example, **antiemetic** drugs that can prevent or reduce nausea and vomiting.

Elderly people seem to be able to tolerate chemotherapy for colorectal cancer. There is no reason to withhold treatment in otherwise healthy people because of age.

Targeted Therapies

Targeted therapies are those that specifically attack some part of cancer cells that make them different from normal cells. Because of this, they should cause fewer side effects than chemotherapy drugs.

Cetuximab (Erbitux) was the first targeted therapy approved for treating colorectal cancer. It is a manmade protein called a monoclonal antibody that specifically attacks the epidermal growth factor receptor (EGFR), a molecule that often appears in high amounts on the surface of cancer cells.

The FDA has approved cetuximab for use with irinotecan or without irinotecan in those who can't take irinotecan or whose cancer is no longer responding to it. In about 10% of patients whose cancers continue to grow despite other treatments, cetuximab will cause tumor shrinkage. This figure is doubled when cetuximab is combined with irinotecan, even if the patients have already been treated with irinotecan and are no longer responding.

Cetuximab is given by intravenous injection. The most serious side effect of cetuximab is an allergic reaction during the first infusion, which could cause problems with breathing and low blood pressure. Other less serious side effects may include an acne-like rash, dry skin, tiredness, fever, and constipation.

Bevacizumab (Avastin), another monoclonal antibody, is approved for first-line use against metastatic colorectal cancer. It is used along with chemotherapy drugs. This antibody is directed against vascular endothelial growth factor (VEGF), a protein that helps tumors form new blood vessels to get nutrients (a process known as angiogenesis). In one study, when bevacizumab was given along with an irinotecan-containing chemotherapy regimen, it increased the shrinkage rate in tumors by 30% over that in patients who were given the same chemotherapy without bevacizumab. It also nearly doubled the time it took for the tumors to grow back. Bevacizumab is the first anti-angiogenesis drug approved to treat colorectal cancer. It is given by intravenous infusion.

Rare but possibly serious side effects include bleeding, holes forming in the colon (requiring surgery to correct), and slow wound healing. More common side effects include high blood pressure, tiredness, blood clots, low white blood cell counts, headaches, mouth sores, loss of appetite, and diarrhea.

Clinical trials are in progress that are testing whether adding either bevacizumab or cetuximab to chemotherapy will further lower the chance of recurrence.

Cost of Drugs

Some of the cancer drugs described are very expensive. 5-FU and leucovorin are inexpensive, but 8 weeks of treatment with a combination that includes oxaliplatin or irinotecan and either bevacizumab or cetuximab will cost at least $20,000 to $30,000. Patients on Medicare without any other insurance will need to pay for 20% of this cost.

Clinical Trials

The purpose of clinical trials

Studies of promising new or experimental treatments in patients are known as **clinical trials**. A clinical trial is only done when there is some reason to believe that the treatment being studied may be valuable to the patient. Treatments used in clinical trials are often found to have real benefits. Researchers conduct studies of new treatments to answer the following questions:

- Is the treatment helpful?
- How does this new type of treatment work?
- Does it work better than other treatments already available?
- What side effects does the treatment cause?
- Are the side effects greater or less than the standard treatment?
- Do the benefits outweigh the side effects?
- In which patients is the treatment most likely to be helpful?

Types of clinical trials

There are 3 phases of clinical trials in which a treatment is studied before it is eligible for approval by the FDA (Food and Drug Administration).

Phase I clinical trials

The purpose of a phase I study is to find the best way to give a new treatment and how much of it can be given safely. The cancer care team watches patients carefully for any harmful side effects. The treatment has been well tested in lab and animal studies, but the side effects in patients are not completely known. Doctors conducting the clinical trial start by giving very low doses of the drug to the first patients and increasing the dose for later groups of patients until side effects appear. Although doctors are hoping to help patients, the main purpose of a phase I study is to test the safety of the drug.

Phase II clinical trials

These studies are designed to see if the drug works. Patients are given the highest dose that doesn't cause severe side effects (determined from the phase I study) and closely observed for an effect on the cancer. The cancer care team also looks for side effects.

Phase III clinical trials

Phase III studies involve large numbers of patients —often several hundred. One group (the control group) receives the standard (most accepted) treatment. The other group receives the new treatment. All patients in phase III studies are closely watched. The study will be stopped if the side effects of the new treatment are too severe or if one group has had much better results than the others.

If you are in a clinical trial, you will have a team of experts taking care of you and monitoring your progress very carefully. The study is especially designed to pay close attention to you.

However, there are some risks. No one involved in the study knows in advance whether the treatment will work or exactly what side effects will occur. That is what the study is designed to find out. While most side effects disappear in time, some can be permanent or even life threatening. Keep in mind, though, that even standard treatments have side effects. Depending on many factors, you may decide to enroll in a clinical trial.

Deciding to enter a clinical trial

Enrollment in any clinical trial is completely up to you. Your doctors and nurses will explain the study to you in detail and will give you a form to read and sign indicating your desire to take part. This process is known as giving your informed consent. Even after signing the form and after the clinical trial begins, you are free to leave the study at any time, for any reason. Taking part in the study does not prevent you from getting other medical care you may need.

To find out more about clinical trials, ask your cancer care team. Among the questions you should ask are:

- Is there a clinical trial for which I would be eligible?
- What is the purpose of the study?
- What kinds of tests and treatments does the study involve?
- What does this treatment do? Has it been used before?
- Will I know which treatment I receive?
- What is likely to happen in my case with, or without, this new treatment?
- What are my other choices and their advantages and disadvantages?

- How could the study affect my daily life?
- What side effects can I expect from the study? Can the side effects be controlled?
- Will I have to be hospitalized? If so, how often and for how long?
- Will the study cost me anything? Will any of the treatment be free?
- If I am harmed as a result of the research, what treatment would I be entitled to?
- What type of long-term follow-up care is part of the study?
- Has the treatment been used to treat other types of cancers?

The American Cancer Society offers a clinical trials matching service for patients, their family, and friends. You can reach this service at 1-800-303-5691 or on our Web site at http://clinicaltrials.cancer.org. Based on the information you provide about your cancer type, stage, and previous treatments, this service can compile a list of clinical trials that match your medical needs. In finding a center most convenient for you, the service can also take into account where you live and whether you are willing to travel.

You can also get a list of current clinical trials by calling the National Cancer Institute's (NCI) Cancer Information Service toll free at 1-800-4-CANCER or by visiting the NCI clinical trials Web site at www.cancer. gov/clinical_trials/.

Treatment by Stage of Colon Cancer

For all but stage IV disease, surgery to remove the colon tumor is the primary or first treatment. **Adjuvant therapy** (additional treatments) may also be used.

Stage 0

Since your cancer has not grown beyond the inner lining of the colon, surgery to take out the cancer is all that is needed. This may be accomplished in many cases by polypectomy or local excision through the colonoscope. Colon resection may be necessary if your tumor is too big to be removed by local excision.

Stage I

Your cancer has grown through several layers of the colon. But it has not spread outside the colon wall itself. Surgical resection to remove the cancer is the standard treatment. You do not need any additional therapy.

Stage II

Your cancer has grown through the wall of the colon and may extend into nearby tissue. It has not yet spread to the lymph nodes. Surgical resection is usually the only treatment you need. If your doctor thinks your cancer is likely to come back because of its appearance under the microscope or because it was growing into other tissues, radiation therapy or chemotherapy may be recommended. Radiation therapy can be given to the area of your abdomen where the cancer was growing. Chemotherapy is not standard treatment for this stage of colon cancer, but many doctors recommend it if the risk of recurrence seems high. There are clinical trials studying this issue, and you might consider enrolling in one. If your doctor recommends chemotherapy, it will likely be the FOLFOX regimen, although some doctors may prefer other regimens such as 5-FU and leucovorin or capecitabine because they are better suited to your health needs.

Stage III

This is a more advanced stage. Your cancer has spread to nearby lymph nodes. But it has not yet spread to other parts of the body. Surgical resection is the first treatment. You should then receive chemotherapy. It will likely be the FOLFOX regimen, although some doctors may prefer other regimens such as 5-FU and leucovorin or capecitabine because they are better suited to your health needs. You may need radiation therapy if your cancer was large enough to grow into adjacent tissues.

Stage IV

In this stage the cancer has spread to distant organs and tissues such as the liver, lungs, peritoneum, or ovaries. The goal of surgery (segmental resection or diverting colostomy) in this stage is usually to relieve or prevent blockage of the colon and to prevent other local complications. In some patients with extensive metastases (spread of cancer), blockage can be prevented or managed by inserting a tube through the tumor (stent) during colonoscopy so that surgery can be avoided. If your cancer is small and your health poor, you might not have surgery.

Surgery in stage IV is usually not done with the expectation of curing the colon cancer. However, if only a few small metastases (usually 5 or fewer) are present in the liver and can be completely removed along with the colon cancer, surgery can help you live longer and may even cure you. You may also be treated with chemotherapy after this. It could be given directly into the arteries that lead into the liver. Another alternative would be intravenous chemotherapy with 5-FU and leucovorin with or without oxaliplatin, the FOLFOX regimen. Recently, doctors have found that adding bevacizumab (Avastin) to this regimen is more effective. Capecitabine pills or irinotecan combined with cetuximab are other alternatives.

If metastases cannot be surgically removed because they are too large or there are too many of them, it may be possible to destroy the tumors by freezing, heating with microwaves, or other nonsurgical methods. Chemotherapy or radiation therapy (or both) may be given to relieve, delay, or prevent symptoms.

Recurrent colon cancer

Recurrent cancer means that your cancer has returned after treatment. The recurrence may be local (near the area of the initial tumor) or it may affect distant organs. Surgery to remove local recurrences can sometimes help you live longer. As with stage IV colon cancer, surgery to remove metastases can also sometimes help you and, along with chemotherapy, can still be curative.

If the metastases can't be removed, chemotherapy with FOLFOX or irinotecan with 5-FU and leucovorin are the main treatments. The FOLFOX may be combined with bevacizumab and the irinotecan with cetuximab. Capecitabine or 5 FU and leucovorin are other options. Drugs are selected based on which, if any, chemotherapy drugs you received before the cancer came back and how long ago you received them. You also might want to discuss appropriate clinical trials with your doctor.

Treatment by Stage of Rectal Cancer

Except for some patients with stage IV cancer, surgery to remove the rectal cancer is the first treatment. **Adjuvant therapy** (additional treatments) may also be used.

Stage 0

At this stage the cancer has not grown beyond the inner lining of the rectum. Removing or destroying the cancer is all that is needed. You can be treated with a **polypectomy**, **local excision**, or **full thickness rectal resection**. You will need no further treatment.

Stage I

In this stage your cancer has grown through the first layer of the rectum into deeper layers but has not spread outside the rectal wall itself. Primary surgery is usually either *low anterior resection* or *abdominoperineal resection*, depending on exactly where the cancer is found within your rectum. Some small stage I rectal cancers may be treated by removing them through the anus without an abdominal incision. You should need no further treatment.

If you are too sick or old to withstand surgery, you may be treated only with radiation therapy. Sometimes this is endocavitary radiation therapy (aiming radiation through the anus) or brachytherapy (placing radioactive pellets directly into the cancer). However, this has not been proven to be as effective as surgery.

Stage II

The cancer has grown through the wall of your rectum into nearby tissue. It has not yet spread to the lymph nodes. Stage II rectal cancers are usually treated by low anterior resection or abdominoperineal resection, along with both chemotherapy and radiation therapy. Radiation can be given either before or after your surgery. Most doctors now favor giving the radiation therapy along with chemotherapy before surgery. Also, many doctors now favor giving adjuvant chemotherapy after surgery. It will likely be the FOLFOX regimen, although some doctors may prefer other regimens such as 5-FU and leucovorin or capecitabine because they are better suited to your health needs.

In some cases of stage II rectal cancer, transanal full thickness rectal resection can be done after chemotherapy and radiation therapy. This approach can prevent the need for abdominoperineal resection and colostomy in some cases. The problem with this is there is no way of knowing whether the cancer has spread to your lymph nodes or being sure the cancer hasn't spread further in your pelvis. Because of this, this procedure isn't generally recommended.

Stage III

Your cancer has spread to nearby lymph nodes but not to other parts of your body. The rectal tumor is usually removed by low anterior resection or abdominoperineal resection. Radiation therapy will be given before or after surgery. As in stage II, many doctors now prefer to give the radiation therapy along with chemotherapy before surgery because it lowers the chance that the cancer will come back in the pelvis. It will also be used for large tumors to make the surgery more effective.

You should then receive chemotherapy. The FOLFOX regimen is the one that many experts recommend. Alternatives are 5-FU and leucovorin or capecitabine, which may better suit their health needs.

Stage IV

Your cancer has spread to distant organs and tissues such as your liver or lungs. The goal of surgery in this stage is to relieve or prevent blockage of your rectum by the cancer and to prevent local complications such as bleeding. Sometimes inserting a tube through the cancer (stent) during colonoscopy can open the blockage. The cancer usually cannot be cured by rectal surgery because it has spread. However, in some cases, it may be possible to remove the rectal tumor, as well as the metastases if only a few are present.

This surgery can help you live longer and/or relieve some of your symptoms. If only a few liver metastases are present, completely removing them along with the rectal tumor may even cure you. If metastases cannot be removed by surgery because they are too large or there are too many of them, it may be possible to destroy the tumors by freezing (cryosurgery), heating with microwaves, photocoagulation (vaporizing the tumor with a laser), or other nonsurgical methods. You may also receive chemotherapy or radiation therapy (or both) to relieve, delay, or prevent symptoms.

It is usually important to treat the rectal tumor with either surgery or radiation therapy, perhaps combined with chemotherapy to prevent blocking of the rectum and/or spread into surrounding tissues. If it appears that the cancer can't be removed or shrunk, then a colostomy will be done to get around any rectal blockage.

If you have only liver metastases, you may be treated with chemotherapy given directly into the artery leading to the liver. This shrinks the cancers in the liver more effectively than if the chemotherapy is given intravenously. If there are only a few liver metastases, removing them with surgery may prolong life and even be curative.

Recurrent rectal cancer

Recurrent cancer means that the cancer has returned after treatment. It may come back locally (near the area of the initial rectal tumor) or in distant organs. Surgery to remove local recurrences can help you live longer. If the tumor cannot be completely removed, combined chemotherapy and radiation therapy may be used. Sometimes, this combination shrinks the cancer enough that complete surgical removal is then possible. If the metastases can't be removed, chemotherapy with FOLFOX or irinotecan along with 5-FU and leucovorin are the main treatments. The FOLFOX may be combined with bevacizumab and the irinotecan/FU/leucovorin with cetuximab. Capecitabine and 5-FU with leucovorin are other options.

Drugs are selected based on which, if any, chemotherapy drugs you received before the cancer came back and how long ago you received them along with your particular health needs. You also might want to discuss with your doctor whether you might enroll in a clinical trial.

Complementary and Alternative Methods

Complementary and alternative therapies are a diverse group of health care practices, systems, and products that are not part of usual medical treatment. They may include products such as vitamins, herbs, or dietary supplements, or procedures such as acupuncture, massage, and a host of other types of treatment. There is a great deal of interest today in complementary and alternative treatments for cancer. Many are now being studied to find out if they are truly helpful to people with cancer.

You may hear about different treatments from family, friends, and others, which may be offered as a way to treat your cancer or to help you feel better. Some of these treatments are harmless in certain situations, while others have been shown to cause harm. Most of them are of unproven benefit.

The American Cancer Society defines **complementary** medicine or methods as those that are used along with your regular medical care. If these treatments are carefully managed, they may add to your comfort and well-being. **Alternative** medicines are defined as those that are used instead of your regular medical care. Some of them have been proven not to be useful or even to be harmful, but are still promoted as "cures." If you choose to use these alternatives, they may reduce your chance of fighting your cancer by delaying, replacing, or interfering with regular cancer treatment.

Before changing your treatment or adding any of these methods, discuss this openly with your doctor or nurse. Some methods can be safely used along with standard medical treatment. Others, however, can interfere with standard treatment or cause serious side effects. That is why it's important to talk with your doctor. More information about specific complementary and alternative therapies used for cancer is available through our toll-free number (1-800-ACS-2345) or on our Web site (www.cancer.org).

More Treatment Information

For more details on treatment options—including some that may not be addressed in this document—the National Comprehensive Cancer Network (NCCN) and the National Cancer Institute (NCI) are good sources of information.

The NCCN, made up of experts from 19 of the nation's leading cancer centers, develops cancer treatment guidelines for doctors to use when treating patients. Those are available on the NCCN Web site (www.nccn.org).

The American Cancer Society collaborates with the NCCN to produce a version of some of these treatment guidelines, written specifically for patients and their families. These less-technical versions are available on both the NCCN Web site (www.nccn.org) and the ACS Web site (www.cancer.org). A print version can also be requested from the ACS at 1-800-ACS-2345.

The NCI provides treatment guidelines via its telephone information center (1-800-4-CANCER) and its Web site (www.cancer.gov). Detailed guidelines intended for use by cancer care professionals are also available on www.cancer.gov.

Questions To Ask

What Should You Ask Your Doctor About Colorectal Cancer?

It is important to have frank, open discussions with your cancer care team. They want to answer all of your questions, so that you can make informed treatment and life decisions. For instance, consider these questions:

- ❏ Where is my cancer located?
- ❏ Has my cancer spread beyond the primary site?
- ❏ What is the stage of my cancer and what does that mean in my case?
- ❏ What treatment choices do I have?
- ❏ What do you recommend and why?
- ❏ What risks or side effects are there to the treatments you suggest? What are the chances my cancer will come back with these treatment plans?
- ❏ What should I do to be ready for treatment?
- ❏ What can I do to reduce the side effects of treatment?
- ❏ Should I follow a special diet?

In addition to these sample questions, be sure to write down some of your own. For instance, you might want more information about recovery times so you can plan your work schedule. Or you may want to ask about second opinions or about clinical trials for which you may qualify.

After Treatment

What Happens After Treatment for Colorectal Cancer?

Completing treatment can be both stressful and exciting. You will be relieved to finish treatment, yet it is hard not to worry about cancer coming back. (When cancer returns, it is called recurrence.) This is a very common concern among those who have had cancer.

It may take a while before your confidence in your own recovery begins to feel real and your fears are somewhat relieved. Even with no recurrences, people who have had cancer learn to live with uncertainty.

Follow-up Care

After your treatment is over, it is very important to keep all follow-up appointments. During these visits, your doctors will ask about symptoms, do physical exams, and order blood tests or imaging studies such as CT scans or x-rays. Follow-up is needed to check for cancer recurrence or spread, as well as possible side effects of certain treatments. This is the time for you to ask your health care team any questions you need answered and to discuss any concerns you might have.

Almost any cancer treatment can have side effects. Some may last for a few weeks to several months, but others can be permanent. Don't hesitate to tell your cancer care team about any symptoms or side effects that bother you so they can help you manage them.

Imaging

Because removing a few liver metastases may be curative, your doctor may want to pay special attention to examining your liver with frequent CT scans or PET scans, especially in the first 2 years after surgery.

Tumor markers

Carcinoembryonic antigen (CEA) and CA 19-9 are substances in the blood of some people with colorectal cancer. Tests for these substances are sometimes useful if you have any symptoms that suggest the cancer has come back. Some doctors perform these tests routinely in order to detect recurrences before you have symptoms. Usually these are most important in the first 2 years after treatment, when most recurrences occur.

For patients with a colostomy

If you have a colostomy, you may feel worried or isolated from normal activities. Whether your ostomy is temporary or permanent, an enterostomal therapist (a health care professional trained to help people with their colostomies) can teach you about the care of your colostomy. You can ask the American Cancer Society about programs offering information and support in your area.

Seeing a new doctor

At some point after your cancer diagnosis and treatment, you may find yourself in the office of a new doctor. Your original doctor may have moved or retired, or you may have moved or changed doctors for some reason. It is important that you be able to give your new doctor the exact details of your diagnosis and treatment. Make sure you have the following information handy:

- a copy of your pathology report from any biopsy or surgery
- if you had surgery, a copy of your operative report
- if you were hospitalized, a copy of the discharge summary that every doctor must prepare when patients are sent home from the hospital
- finally, since some cancer treatment drugs can have long-term side effects, a list of your drugs, drug doses, and when you took them

Lifestyle Changes to Consider During and After Treatment

Having cancer and dealing with treatment can be time-consuming and emotionally draining, but it can also be a time to look at your life in new ways. Maybe you are thinking about how to improve your health over the long term. Some people even begin this process during cancer treatment.

Make healthier choices

Think about your life before you learned you had cancer. Were there things you did that might have made you less healthy? Maybe you drank too much alcohol, or ate more than you needed, or smoked, or didn't exercise very often. Emotionally, maybe you kept your feelings bottled up, or maybe you let stressful situations go on too long.

Now is not the time to feel guilty or to blame yourself. However, you can start making changes *today* that can have positive effects for the rest of your life. Not only will you feel better but you will also be healthier. What better time than now to take advantage of the motivation you have as a result of going through a life-changing experience like having cancer?

You can start by working on those things that you feel most concerned about. Get help with those that are harder for you. For instance, if you are thinking about quitting smoking and need help, call our Quitline at 1-800-ACS-2345.

Diet and nutrition

Eating right can be a challenge for anyone, but it can get even tougher during and after cancer treatment. For instance, treatment often may change your sense of taste. Nausea can be a problem. You may lose your appetite for a while and lose weight when you don't want to. On the other hand, some people gain weight even without eating more. This can be frustrating, too.

If you are losing weight or have taste problems during treatment, do the best you can with eating and remember that these problems usually improve over time. You may want to ask your cancer team for a referral to a dietitian, an expert in nutrition who can give you ideas on how to fight some of the side effects of your treatment. You may also find it helps to eat small portions every 2 to 3 hours until you feel better and can go back to a more normal schedule.

One of the best things you can do after treatment is to put healthy eating habits into place. You will be surprised at the long-term benefits of some simple changes, like increasing the variety of healthy foods you eat. Try to eat 5 or more servings of vegetables and fruits each day. Choose whole grain foods instead of white flour and sugars. Try to limit meats that are high in fat. Cut back on processed meats like hot dogs, bologna, and bacon. Get rid of them altogether if you can. If you drink alcohol, limit yourself to 1 or 2 drinks a day at the most. And don't forget to get some type of regular exercise. The combination of a good diet and regular exercise will help you maintain a healthy weight and keep you feeling more energetic.

Rest, fatigue, work, and exercise

Fatigue is a very common symptom in people being treated for cancer. This is often not an ordinary type of tiredness but a "bone-weary" exhaustion that doesn't get better with rest. For some, this fatigue lasts a long time after treatment, and can discourage them from physical activity.

However, exercise can actually help you reduce fatigue. Studies have shown that patients who follow an exercise program tailored to their personal needs feel physically and emotionally improved and can cope better.

If you are ill and need to be on bed rest during treatment, it is normal to expect your fitness, endurance, and muscle strength to decline some. Physical therapy can help you maintain strength and range of motion in your muscles, which can help fight fatigue and the sense of depression that sometimes comes with feeling so tired.

Any program of physical activity should fit your own situation. An older person who has never exercised will not be able to take on the same amount of exercise as a 20-year-old who plays tennis 3 times a week. If you haven't exercised in a few years but can still get around, you may want to think about taking short walks.

Talk with your health care team before starting, and get their opinion about your exercise plans. Then, try to get an exercise buddy so that you're not doing it alone. Having family or friends involved when starting a new exercise program can give you that extra boost of support to keep you going when the push just isn't there.

If you are very tired, though, you will need to balance activity with rest. It is okay to rest when you need to. It is really hard for some people to allow themselves to do that when they are used to working all day or taking care of a household.

Exercise can improve your physical and emotional health:

- It improves your cardiovascular (heart and circulation) fitness.
- It strengthens your muscles.
- It reduces fatigue.
- It lowers anxiety and depression.
- It makes you feel generally happier.
- It helps you feel better about yourself.

And long term, we know that exercise plays a role in preventing some cancers. The American Cancer Society, in its guidelines on physical activity for cancer prevention, recommends that adults take part in at least 1 physical activity for 30 minutes or more on 5 days or more of the week. Children and teens are encouraged to try for at least 60 minutes a day of energetic physical activity on at least 5 days a week.

How About Your Emotional Health?

Once your treatment ends, you may find yourself overwhelmed by emotions. This happens to a lot of people. You may have been going through so much during treatment that you could only focus on getting through your treatment.

Now you may find that you think about the potential of your own death, or the effect of your cancer on your family, friends, and career. You may also begin to re-evaluate your relationship with your spouse or partner. Unexpected issues may also cause concern— for instance, as you become healthier and have fewer doctor visits, you will see your health care team less often. That can be a source of anxiety for some.

This is an ideal time to seek out emotional and social support. You need people you can turn to for strength and comfort. Support can come in many forms: family, friends, cancer support groups, church or spiritual groups, online support communities, or individual counselors.

Almost everyone who has been through cancer can benefit from getting some type of support. What's best for you depends on your situation and personality. Some people feel safe in peer-support groups or education groups. Others would rather talk in an informal setting, such as church. Others may feel more at ease talking one-on-one with a trusted friend or counselor. Whatever your source of strength or comfort, make sure you have a place to go with your concerns.

The cancer journey can feel very lonely. It is not necessary or realistic to go it all by yourself. And your friends and family may feel shut out if you decide not to include them. Let them in—and let in anyone else who you feel may help. If you aren't sure who can help, call your American Cancer Society at 1-800-ACS-2345 and we can put you in touch with an appropriate group or resource.

You can't change the fact that you have had cancer. What you can change is how you live the rest of your life—making healthy choices and feeling as well as possible, physically and emotionally.

What Happens If Treatment Is No Longer Working?

If cancer continues to grow after one kind of treatment, or if it returns, it is often possible to try another treatment plan that might still cure the cancer, or at least shrink the tumors enough to help you live longer and feel better. On the other hand, when a person has received several different medical treatments and the cancer has not been cured, over time the cancer tends to become resistant to all treatment. At this time it's important to weigh the possible limited benefit of a new treatment against the possible downsides, including continued doctor visits and treatment side effects.

Everyone has his or her own way of looking at this. Some people may want to focus on remaining comfortable during their limited time left.

This is likely to be the most difficult time in your battle with cancer—when you have tried everything medically within reason and it's just not working anymore. Although your doctor may offer you new treatment, you need to consider that at some point, continuing treatment is not likely to improve your health or change your prognosis or survival.

If you want to continue treatment to fight your cancer as long as you can, you still need to consider the odds of more treatment having any benefit. In many cases, your doctor can estimate the response rate for the treatment you are considering. Some people are tempted to try more chemotherapy or radiation, for example, even when their doctors say that the odds of benefit are less than 1%. In this situation, you need to think about and understand your reasons for choosing this plan.

No matter what you decide to do, it is important that you be as comfortable as possible. Make sure you are asking for and getting treatment for any symptoms you might have, such as pain. This type of treatment is called "palliative" treatment.

Palliative treatment helps relieve these symptoms, but is not expected to cure the disease; its main purpose is to improve your quality of life. Sometimes, the treatments you get to control your symptoms are similar to the treatments used to treat cancer. For example, radiation therapy might be given to help relieve bone pain from bone metastasis. Or chemotherapy might be given to help shrink a tumor and keep it from causing a bowel obstruction. But this is not the same as receiving treatment to try to cure the cancer.

At some point, you may benefit from hospice care. Most of the time, this can be given at home. Your cancer may be causing symptoms or problems that need attention, and hospice focuses on your comfort. You should know that receiving hospice care doesn't mean you can't have treatment for the problems caused by your cancer or other health conditions. It just means that the focus of your care is on living life as fully as possible and feeling as well as you can at this difficult stage of your cancer.

Remember also that maintaining hope is important. Your hope for a cure may not be as bright, but there is still hope for good times with family and friends—times that are filled with happiness and meaning. In a way, pausing at this time in your cancer treatment is an opportunity to refocus on the most important things in your life. This is the time to do some things you've always wanted to do and to stop doing the things you no longer want to do.

Latest Research

What's New in Colorectal Cancer Research and Treatment?

Research is always under way in the area of colorectal cancer. Scientists are looking for causes and ways to prevent colorectal cancer as well as ways to improve treatments.

Chemoprevention

Chemoprevention is the use of natural or man-made chemicals to lower a person's risk of developing cancer. Researchers are testing whether fiber supplements, minerals (such as calcium), and vitamins can lower colorectal cancer risk. Some studies have found that people who take multivitamins containing folic acid (also known as folate) have a lower colorectal cancer risk than people who do not. Studies of vitamin A, C, D, and E supplements have yielded conflicting results. But recent studies have found that people who took vitamin D supplements had a reduced rate of colorectal cancer. Increasing calcium intake by using calcium supplements or eating extra amounts of low-fat dairy products may reduce formation of colorectal adenomatous polyps.

Although taking aspirin or some other non-steroidal anti-inflammatory drugs (NSAIDS) is associated with a lower risk of colorectal cancer, these drugs can cause stomach ulcers and other side effects. For this reason, taking NSAIDS specifically for this purpose is not recommended for people at average colorectal cancer risk.

NSAIDs, such as sulindac and celecoxib (Celebrex), have been shown to reduce formation of adenomatous polyps in people with familial adenomatous polyposis (FAP). The FDA has recently approved celecoxib for reducing polyp formation in people with FAP. However, recent celecoxib data are now being evaluated for a potential increased heart risk.

Studies indicate that a diet high in fruits and vegetables may lower colorectal cancer risk, as well as the risk of several other diseases. This hasn't been completely proven by all studies. Nearly all experts, however, agree fiber supplements alone are not as beneficial as getting dietary fiber by eating foods from plant sources. But it is important that you eat enough servings—at least 5 a day!

Most experts recommend that people not take large doses of vitamins, minerals, or other agents unless they are part of a study or are under the advice and care of a doctor.

Genetics

Scientists are learning more about some of the inherited and acquired changes in DNA that cause cells of the colon and rectum to become cancerous. Recent discoveries of inherited genes that increase a person's risk of developing colorectal cancer are already being used in genetic tests to inform people most at risk.

Advances in understanding how these genes work are expected to eventually lead to new drugs and gene therapies to correct these gene problems. Early phases of gene therapy trials are already in progress. Researchers have developed ways to package DNA of normal p53 genes into a virus designed in the laboratory. Most colorectal cancer cells have defects of this tumor suppressor gene that contribute to their abnormal growth and spread. Studies are under way to see whether these designer viruses containing normal p53 genes can infect colorectal cancer cells and either stop their growth or cause them to "self-destruct."

Earlier detection

Studies continue to evaluate the effectiveness of current colorectal cancer screening methods and evaluate new approaches to informing the public about the importance of taking advantage of these methods. Less than half of Americans older than age 50 have any colorectal cancer screening at all. If everyone were tested, tens of thousands of lives could be saved each year. The American Cancer Society and other public health organizations are working to increase awareness of colorectal cancer screening among the general public and health care professionals. Meanwhile, new imaging and laboratory tests are also being developed and tested.

Researchers know of DNA mutations that often affect certain genes (such as the APC gene, K-ras oncogene, and p53 tumor suppressor gene) in colorectal cancer cells. Studies are testing new ways to recognize these DNA mutations in cells found in stool samples, to see if this screening approach is useful in finding large polyps and colorectal cancers at an earlier stage.

Cells from the lining layer of the colon and rectum are constantly shed into the stool and replaced by new cells. The cells that slough off the lining typically undergo apoptosis, a specific type of cell death that causes recognizable changes in the cells' DNA. Cells that slough off from the surface of colon cancers do not usually undergo these changes. Finding intact-appearing DNA (that lacks the changes of apoptosis) in stool samples appears to be useful in finding colorectal cancers. Recent studies that have combined DNA tests to look for gene mutations and for intact-appearing DNA have shown promising results. Nonetheless, more research is needed to confirm the accuracy of these tests before widespread use can be recommended.

Virtual colonoscopy is a special type of CT scan that can find colorectal polyps and cancers at least as accurately as a barium enema. This test is described in more detail in the section, "Can Colorectal Polyps and Cancer Be Found Early?" (See page 24.)

Although virtual colonoscopy is currently not included among the tests recommended by American Cancer Society for early detection of colorectal cancer, the Society is carefully following progress in this area as technology improves and more results become available about its accuracy.

Immunotherapy

Experimental treatments that boost the patient's immune reaction to fight colorectal cancer more effectively are being tested in clinical trials. Some treatments use drugs like interferons and interleukins that boost the immune system in general.

In active immunotherapy, the patient is given a vaccine that might cause the immune system to recognize some of the abnormal chemicals in colorectal cancer cells and kill these cells. For example, the K-ras oncogene product is altered in many colorectal cancers and researchers are testing ways to help the patient's immune system attack cells with an altered ras protein. Researchers are also testing vaccines to direct a patient's immune system to attack colorectal cancer cells that produce carcinoembryonic antigen (CEA). There are also studies where patients' tumor cells are used to produce a vaccine. The vaccine is used for adjuvant therapy in the hope of preventing recurrence.

Passive immunotherapy uses antibodies made in the laboratory and then injected into patients to seek out colorectal cancer cells that contain abnormal ras protein or other abnormal or overproduced proteins like carcinoembryonic antigen (CEA) or the HER-2 oncogene product. Toxins or radioactive atoms can be attached to these antibodies, so that the cell-killing chemicals or radiation is targeted specifically to the cancer cells and do not attack the healthy cells of the body. Two antibodies, cetuximab (Erbitux) and bevacizumab (Avastin), are discussed previously in the tumor growth factor section.

Tumor growth factors

Researchers have discovered naturally occurring substances in the body that promote cell growth. These hormone-like substances are called **growth factors**. Growth factors activate cells by attaching to growth factor receptors, which are present on the outer surface of the cells. Some cancer cells grow especially fast because they contain more growth factor receptors than normal cells do. One of the growth factors that has been linked to colorectal cancers is called **epidermal growth factor** (EGF).

New drugs like cetuximab (Erbitux) that specifically kill cancer cells by attacking EGF receptors have proven effective and are now being used. More are being developed.

Another growth factor, known as **vascular endothelial growth factor** (VEGF), helps tumors develop new blood vessels to get nutrients. Several drugs are now in development to try to block VEGF in order to cut off the tumor's blood supply. These drugs are known as **antiangiogenesis** drugs.

One such drug, bevacizumab (Avastin), is a monoclonal antibody that attacks VEGF. This has proven effective also and is now being used to treat colorectal cancer. Other drugs that act against blood vessels are being developed and tested.

Chemotherapy

Many clinical trials are testing new chemotherapy drugs or drugs that are now used against other cancers (such as cisplatin or gemcitabine). Other studies are looking at ways to combine drugs already known to be active against colorectal cancer, such as irinotecan or oxaliplatin, to improve their effectiveness. Still other studies are testing the best ways to combine chemotherapy with radiation therapy or immunotherapy.

Resources

Additional Resources

More Information From Your American Cancer Society

We have selected some related information that may also be helpful to you. These materials may be viewed on our Web site or ordered from our toll-free number, 1-800-ACS-2345.

> *After Diagnosis: A Guide for Patients and Families* (also available in Spanish)

> *ACS/NCCN Colon and Rectal Cancer: Treatment Guidelines for Patients*

> *Nutrition for the Person With Cancer: A Guide for Patients and Families* (also available in Spanish)

> *Colostomy – A Guide* (also available in Spanish)

> *Sexuality & Cancer: For the Man Who Has Cancer and His Partner* (also available in Spanish)

> *Sexuality & Cancer: For the Woman Who Has Cancer and Her Partner* (also available in Spanish)

The following books are available from the American Cancer Society. Call us at 1-800-ACS-2345 to ask about costs or to place your order.

> *American Cancer Society's Consumer Guide to Cancer Drugs*, Second Edition

American Cancer Society's Complete Guide to Colorectal Cancer

American Cancer Society's Guide to Pain Control: Understanding and Managing Cancer Pain, Revised Edition

Because... Someone I Love Has Cancer: Kids' Activity Book

Cancer in the Family: Helping Children Cope With a Parent's Illness

Cancer: What Causes It, What Doesn't

Caregiving: A Step-By-Step Resource for Caring for the Person With Cancer at Home, Revised Edition

Coming to Terms With Cancer: A Glossary of Cancer-Related Terms

Couples Confronting Cancer: Keeping Your Relationship Strong

Eating Well, Staying Well During and After Cancer

Informed Decisions: The Complete Book of Cancer Diagnosis, Treatment, and Recovery, Second Edition

Lymphedema: Understanding and Managing Lymphedema After Cancer Treatment

Our Mom Has Cancer

When the Focus Is on Care: Palliative Care and Cancer

National Organizations and Web Sites

In addition to the American Cancer Society, other sources of patient information and support include*:

American College of Gastroenterology
Internet Address: www.acg.gi.org

American Gastroenterological Association
Telephone: 1-301-654-2055
Internet Address: www.gastro.org

American Society of Colon and Rectal Surgeons
Internet Address: www.fascrs.org

Colon Cancer Alliance
Telephone: 1-877-422-2030
Internet Address: www.ccalliance.org

Colorectal Cancer Network
Internet Address: www.colorectal-cancer.net/
colorectal.htm

National Cancer Institute
Telephone 1-800-4-CANCER or 1-800-422-6237;
TTY: 1-800-332-8615
Internet Addresses: www.cancer.gov

National Colorectal Cancer Research Alliance
Internet Address: www.eif.nccra.org

Inclusion on this list does not imply endorsement by the American Cancer Society.

The American Cancer Society is happy to address almost any cancer-related topic. If you have any more questions, please call us at 1-800-ACS-2345 at any time, 24 hours a day.

References

American Cancer Society. *Cancer Facts and Figures 2006.* Atlanta, GA: American Cancer Society: 2006.

American Joint Committee on Cancer. Colon and Rectum. In: *AJCC Cancer Staging Manual.* 6th ed. New York: Springer; 2002:113-124.

Levin B, Brooks D, Smith RA, Stone A. Emerging technologies in screening for colorectal cancer. *CA Cancer J Clin.* 2003;53:44-55.

Lynch HT, de la Chapelle A. Hereditary colorectal cancer. *N Engl J Med.* 2003;348:919-932.

National Comprehensive Cancer Network. Colon/rectal cancer. www.nccn.org. Accessed December 2004.

Niederhuber JE, Cole CE, Grochow L, et al. Colon cancer. In: Abeloff MD, Armitage JO, Lichter AS, Niederhuber JE. Kastan MB, McKenna WG, eds. *Clinical Oncology*. Philadelphia, PA. Elsevier: 2004: 1877-1941.

O'Connell JB, Maggard MA, Ko CY. Colon cancer survival rates with the new American Joint Committee on Cancer Sixth Edition staging. *J Natl Cancer Inst.* 2004;96:1420-1425.

Regine WF, Hanna N, DeSimone P, Cohen AM. Cancer of the rectum. In: Abeloff MD, Armitage JO, Lichter AS, Niederhuber JE. Kastan MB, McKenna WG, eds. *Clinical Oncology*. Philadelphia, PA. Elsevier: 2004:1942-1965.

Rodriguez-Bigas MA, Lin EH, Crane CH. Adenocarcinoma of the colon and rectum. In: Kufe DW, Pollock RE, Weichselbaum RR, Bast RC, Gansler TS, Holland JF, Frei E, eds. *Cancer Medicine 6*. Hamilton, Ont: BC Decker; 2003:1635-1666.

Skibber JM, Hoff PM, Minsky BD. Cancer of the rectum. In: DeVita VT, Heilman S, Rosenberg SA, eds. *Cancer: Principles and Practice of Oncology*. Philadelphia, PA: Lippincott Williams & Wilkins; 2001:1271-1312.

Skibber JM, Minsky BD, Hoff PM. Cancer of the colon. In: DeVita VT, Heilman S, Rosenberg SA, eds. *Cancer: Principles and Practice of Oncology*. Philadelphia, PA: Lippincott Williams & Wilkins; 2001:1216-1270.

Umar A, Boland CR, Terdiman JP, et al. Revised Bethesda guidelines for hereditary nonpolyposis colorectal cancer (Lynch syndrome) and microsatellite instability. *J Natl Cancer Inst.* 2004;96:261-268.

Dictionary

Colorectal Cancer Dictionary

abdomen: the part of the body between the chest and the pelvis; it contains the stomach (with the lower part of the esophagus), small and large intestines, liver, gallbladder, spleen, pancreas, and bladder.

adenocarcinoma: cancer of the glandular cells; for example, those that line the inside of the colon and rectum.

adenomatous polyp or **adenoma**: a benign (non-cancerous) growth of glandular cells; for example, those that line the inside of the colon or rectum. There are 3 types of colorectal adenomas: **tubular**, **villous**, and **tuberovillous**.

adjuvant therapy: treatment used in addition to the main treatment. It usually refers to chemotherapy, hormonal therapy, immunotherapy, or radiation therapy added after surgery to increase the chances of curing the cancer or keeping it in check.

advanced cancer: a general term describing stages of cancer in which the disease has spread from the primary site to other parts of the body. When the cancer has spread only to the surrounding areas, it is called **locally advanced**. If it has spread to distant parts of the body, it is called **metastatic**.

advance directives: legal documents that tell the doctor and family what a person wants for future medical care, including whether to start or when to stop life-sustaining treatment.

AJCC Staging System: American Joint Committee on Cancer staging system (also called the TNM system), which describes the extent of a cancer's spread in Roman numerals from 0 through IV. *See also*, **staging**.

alopecia: hair loss, a condition that often results from chemotherapy or from radiation therapy to the head. In most cases, the hair grows back after treatment ends.

alternative therapy: an unproven therapy used instead of standard (proven) therapy. Some alternative therapies may have dangerous or even life-threatening side effects. For others, the main danger is that a patient may lose the opportunity to benefit from standard therapy. The ACS recommends that patients considering use of any alternative or complementary therapy discuss this with their health care team. *See also*, **complementary therapy**.

anastomosis: the site where two structures are surgically joined together.

anesthesia: the loss of feeling or sensation as a result of drugs or gases. General anesthesia causes loss of consciousness (makes you go into a deep sleep). Local or regional anesthesia numbs only a certain area of the body.

angiogenesis: the formation of new blood vessels. Some cancer treatments work by blocking angiogenesis, thus preventing blood from reaching the tumor.

anorexia: loss of appetite; may be caused by either the cancer itself or as a side effect of treatments such as chemotherapy.

antibody: a protein produced by the body's immune system cells and released into the blood. Antibodies defend the body against foreign agents, such as bacteria. These agents contain certain substances called antigens. Each antibody works against a specific antigen. *See also*, **antigen**.

antiemetic: a drug that prevents or relieves nausea and vomiting, common side effects of chemotherapy.

antigen: a substance that causes the body's immune system to react. This reaction often involves production of antibodies. For example, the immune system's response to antigens that are part of bacteria and viruses helps people resist infections. Cancer cells have certain antigens that can be found by laboratory tests. They are important in cancer diagnosis and in watching response to treatment. Other cancer cell antigens play a role in immune reactions that may help the body's resistance against cancer.

anus: the outlet of the digestive tract through which stool passes out of the body.

ascending colon: the first of the four sections of the colon. It extends upward on the right side of the abdomen.

Astler-Collier staging system: one of the staging systems for colorectal cancer. In this system, the letters A through D are used for the various stages.

barium sulfate: a chalky liquid used to outline the digestive tract for x-rays. It can be taken by mouth (as part of an upper GI series) or infused through the rectum as a barium enema (as part of a lower GI series).

benign: not cancer; not malignant.

biopsy: the removal of a sample of tissue to see whether cancer cells are present. There are several kinds of biopsies. In an endoscopic biopsy, a small sample of tissue is removed using instruments operated through a colonoscope.

bone scan: an imaging test that gives important information about the bones, including the location of cancer that may have spread to the bones. It can be done on an outpatient basis and is painless, except for the needle stick when a low-dose radioactive substance is injected into a vein. Pictures are taken to see where the radioactivity collects, pointing to an abnormality.

brachytherapy: internal radiation treatment given by placing radioactive material directly into the tumor or close to it. Also called **interstitial radiation therapy** or **seed implantation**.

bowel: the intestine.

CT colonography: *see* **virtual colonoscopy**.

CT scan: *see* **computed tomography**.

cancer: cancer is not just one disease but rather a group of diseases. All forms of cancer cause cells in the body to change and grow out of control. Most types of cancer cells form a lump or mass called a tumor. The tumor can invade and destroy healthy tissue. Cells from the tumor can break away and travel to other parts of the body. There they can continue to grow. This spreading process is called metastasis. When cancer spreads, it is still named after the part of the body where it started. For example, if colorectal cancer spreads to the liver, it is still colorectal cancer, not liver cancer.

Some cancers, such as blood cancers, do not form a tumor. Not all tumors are cancer. A tumor that is not cancer is called **benign**. Benign tumors do not grow and spread the way cancer does. They are usually not a threat to life. Another word for cancerous is **malignant**.

cancer care team: the group of health care professionals who work together to find, treat, and care for people with cancer. The cancer care team may include any or all of the following and others: primary care physicians, pathologists, oncology specialists (medical oncologist, radiation oncologist), surgeons (including surgical specialists such as urologists, gynecologists, neurosurgeons, etc.), nurses, oncology nurse specialists, and oncology social workers. Whether the team is linked formally or informally, there is usually one person who takes the job of coordinating the team.

cancer cell: a cell that divides and reproduces abnormally and can spread throughout the body. *See also,* **metastasis**.

cancer-related checkup: a routine health examination for cancer in persons without obvious signs or symptoms of cancer. The goal of the cancer-related checkup is to find the disease, if it exists, at an early stage, when chances for cure are greatest. Depending on the person's sex and age, this checkup may include a digital rectal examination, clinical breast examinations, Pap smears, PSA blood test, and skin examinations. *See also*, **detection**.

carcinogen: any substance that causes cancer or helps cancer grow. For example, tobacco smoke contains many carcinogens that greatly increase the risk of lung cancer.

carcinoembryonic antigen (CEA): a substance normally found in fetal tissue. If found in an adult it may suggest that a cancer, especially one starting in the digestive system, may be present. Tests for this substance may help in finding out if a colorectal cancer has recurred after treatment.

carcinoma: a malignant tumor that begins in the lining layer (epithelial cells) of organs. At least 80% of all cancers are carcinomas.

carcinoid tumors or carcinoids: tumors that develop from neuroendocrine cells, usually in the digestive tract, lung, or ovary. The cancer cells from these tumors release certain hormones into the bloodstream. In about 10% of people, the hormone levels are high enough to cause facial flushing, wheezing, diarrhea, a fast heartbeat, and other symptoms throughout the body.

cell: the basic unit of which all living things are made. Cells replace themselves by splitting and forming new cells (mitosis). The processes that control the formation of new cells and the death of old cells are disrupted in cancer.

cGy: short for centigray, a unit of radiation equal to the rad, an older term.

chemotherapy: treatment with drugs to destroy cancer cells. Chemotherapy is often used, either alone or with surgery or radiation, to treat cancer that has spread or come back (recurred), or when there is a strong chance that it could recur.

chyme: the thick, nearly liquid mixture of partly digested food and digestive juices found in the stomach and small intestine.

clinical trials: research studies to test new drugs or other treatments to compare current, standard treatments with others that may be better. Before a new treatment is used on people, it is studied in the lab. If lab studies suggest the treatment will work, the next step is to test its value for patients. These human studies are called clinical trials. The main questions the researchers want to answer are:

- Does this treatment work?
- Does it work better than what we're now using?
- What side effects does it cause?
- Do the benefits outweigh the risks?
- Which patients are most likely to find this treatment helpful?

colectomy: surgical removal of all (total colectomy) or part (partial colectomy or hemicolectomy) of the colon.

colitis: a general term for inflammation of the large intestine (colon). Colitis is usually either intermittent or chronic (as in ulcerative colitis).

colon: the large intestine. The colon is a muscular tube about 5 feet long. It is divided into 4 sections: the ascending, transverse, descending, and sigmoid colon. It continues the process of absorbing water and mineral nutrients from food that was started in the small intestine.

colonoscope: a slender, flexible, hollow lighted tube about the thickness of a finger. It is inserted through the rectum up into the colon. A colonoscope is much longer than a sigmoidoscope, and allows the doctor to see much more of the colon's lining. The colonoscope is connected to a video camera and video display monitor so the doctor can look closely at the inside of your colon. (This procedure is called a colonoscopy.)

colorectal cancer: since colon cancer and rectal cancer have many features in common they are sometimes referred to together as colorectal cancer.

colostomy: a procedure in which the end of the colon is attached to an opening created in the abdominal wall to get rid of body waste (stool). A colostomy is sometimes needed after surgery for cancer of the rectum. People with colon cancer sometimes have a temporary colostomy but they rarely need a permanent one.

complementary therapy: therapy used in addition to standard therapy. Some complementary therapies may help relieve certain symptoms of cancer, relieve side effects of standard cancer therapy, or improve a patient's sense of well-being. The ACS recommends that patients considering the use of any alternative or complementary therapy discuss this with their health care team. *See also*, **alternative therapy**.

computed tomography (CT): an imaging test in which many x-ray images are taken from different angles of a part of the body. These images are combined by a computer to produce cross-sectional pictures of internal organs. Except for the injection of a dye (needed in some but not all cases), this is a painless procedure that can be done in an outpatient clinic. It is often referred to as a "CT" or "CAT" scan.

Crohn's disease (Crohn's colitis): a type of chronic inflammatory bowel disease. In this condition, the small bowel or, less often, the colon is inflamed over a long period of time. This increases a person's risk of developing colon cancer, so starting colorectal cancer screening earlier and doing these tests more often is recommended. *See also* **inflammatory bowel disease**.

CT colonography: *see* **virtual colonoscopy**.

curative treatment: treatment aimed at producing a cure. Compare with palliative treatment.

cytology: the branch of science that deals with the structure and function of cells. Also refers to tests to diagnose cancer and other diseases by examination of cells under the microscope.

cytotoxic: toxic to cells; cell-killing.

DNA (deoxyribonucleic acid): the genetic "blueprint" found in the nucleus of each cell. DNA holds genetic information on cell growth, division, and function.

DRE: *see* **digital rectal examination**.

descending colon: the third section of the colon; it continues downward on the left side of the abdomen.

detection: finding disease. Early detection means that the disease is found at an early stage, before it has grown large or spread to other sites. Note: many forms of cancer can reach an advanced stage without causing symptoms.

diagnosis: identifying a disease by its signs or symptoms, and by using imaging procedures and laboratory findings. For some types of cancer, the earlier a diagnosis is made, the better the chance for long-term survival.

dietary supplement: a product, such as a vitamin, mineral, or herb, intended to improve health but not to diagnose, treat, cure, or prevent disease. Because dietary supplements are not considered "drugs," their manufacturers do not have to prove they are effective, or even safe.

differentiation: the normal process through which cells mature so they can carry out the jobs they were meant to do. Cancer cells are less differentiated than normal cells. Pathologists use grading to evaluate and report the degree of a cancer's differentiation.

digestive system: the collection of organs (also called the gastrointestinal tract, or GI tract) that processes food for energy and rids the body of solid waste matter.

digital rectal examination (DRE): an exam during which the doctor inserts a lubricated, gloved finger into the rectum to feel for anything not normal. This simple test, which is not painful, can detect many rectal cancers.

disease-free survival rate: the percentage of people with a certain cancer who still have no evidence of disease (cancer) a certain period of time (usually 5 years) after treatment. This rate does not measure actual "survival," which is expressed by the 5-year survival rate.

double contrast barium enema (DCBE): a method used to help diagnose colorectal cancer. Barium sulfate, a chalky substance, is infused through the rectum to partially fill and open up the colon. When the colon is about half-full of barium, air is inserted to cause the colon to expand. This allows x-ray films to show abnormalities of the colon. Also called barium enema with air contrast.

doubling time: the time it takes for a cell to divide and double itself. Cancers vary in doubling time from 8 to 600 days, averaging 100 to 120 days. Thus, a cancer may be present for many years before it can be felt.

Dukes staging system: one of the staging systems for colorectal cancer, it uses the letters A through C.

dysplasia: abnormal changes of groups of cells that may lead to cancer.

electrofulguration: a type of treatment that destroys cancer cells by burning with an electrical current. Also known as **electrocautery**.

enterostomal therapist: a health professional, often a nurse, who teaches people how to care for ostomies (surgically created openings such as a colostomy) and other wounds.

epidemiology: the study of diseases in populations by collecting and analyzing statistical data. In the field of cancer, epidemiologists look at how many people have cancer; who gets specific types of cancer; and what factors (such as environment, job hazards, family patterns, and personal habits, such as smoking and diet) play a part in the development of cancer.

etiology: the cause of a disease. There are probably many causes of cancer, and research is showing that both genetics and lifestyle are major factors in many cancers.

external beam radiation therapy (EBRT): radiation that is focused from a source outside the body on the area affected by the cancer. It is much like getting a diagnostic x-ray, but for a longer time.

false negative: test result implying a condition does not exist when in fact it does.

false positive: test result implying a condition exists when in fact it does not.

familial adenomatous polyposis (FAP): an inherited condition that is a risk factor for colorectal cancer. People with this syndrome typically develop hundreds of polyps in the colon and rectum. Usually one or more of these polyps becomes cancerous if preventive surgery is not done.

fecal occult blood test (FOBT): a test for "hidden" blood in the feces (stool). The presence of such blood could be a sign of cancer.

feces: solid waste matter; stool.

fiber: dietary fiber includes a wide variety of plant carbo-hydrates that are not digested by humans. Fibers are classified as "soluble" (like oat bran) and "insoluble" (like wheat bran). Soluble fiber helps to reduce blood cholesterol, thereby lowering the risk of heart disease. Good sources of fiber are beans, vegetables, whole grains, and fruits. Links between fiber and cancer risk are inconclusive, but eating these foods is still recommended because they contain other substances that can help prevent cancer and because they have other health benefits.

fine needle aspiration (FNA) biopsy: a procedure in which a thin needle is used to draw up (aspirate) samples for examination under a microscope. FNA is not generally used for biopsies of a colorectal tumor, but is often used to take samples of masses in the liver or other organs that might be colorectal cancer metastases.

five (5)-year survival rate: the percentage of people with a given cancer who are expected to survive 5 years or longer with the disease. Five-year survival rates have some drawbacks. Although the rates are based on the most recent information available, they may include data from patients treated several years earlier. Advances in cancer treatment often occur quickly. Five-year survival rates, while statistically valid, may not reflect these advances.

They should not be seen as a predictor in an individual case. *See also,* **5-year relative survival rate**.

flexible sigmoidoscopy: *see* **sigmoidoscope**.

frozen section: a very thin slice of body tissue that has been quick-frozen and then examined under a microscope. This method is sometimes used during an operation because it gives a quick diagnosis, and can tell a surgeon whether or not to continue with the procedure. The diagnosis is confirmed in a few days by a more detailed study called a permanent section.

Gardner syndrome: like FAP, Gardner syndrome is an inherited condition that results in polyps that develop at a young age and often lead to cancer. It can also cause benign (not cancerous) tumors of the skin, soft connective tissue, and bones.

gastroenterologist: a doctor who specializes in diseases of the digestive (gastrointestinal) tract.

gastrointestinal stromal tumors (GISTs): rare tumors of the connective tissue in the wall of the small intestine, colon, and rectum.

gastrointestinal (GI) tract: the digestive tract. It consists of those organs and structures that process and prepare food to be used for energy; for example, the stomach, small intestine and large intestine.

gene: a segment of DNA that contains information on hereditary characteristics such as hair color, eye color, and height, as well as susceptibility to certain diseases.

grade: the grade of a cancer reflects how abnormal it looks under the microscope. There are several grading systems for different types of cancers. Each grading system divides cancer into those with the greatest abnormality, the least abnormality, and those in between.

Grading is done by a pathologist who examines the tissue from the biopsy. It is important because cancers with more abnormal-appearing cells tend to grow and spread more quickly and have a worse prognosis (outlook).

guaiac test: another name for a fecal occult blood test (FOBT). Guaiac is the substance that can interact with and detect very small amounts of blood in the stool. Hemoccult is a brand of guaiac test.

hemicolectomy: surgical removal of part of the colon.

hereditary nonpolyposis colon cancer (HNPCC): an inherited condition that increases a person's risk for developing colorectal cancer. People with this condition tend to develop cancer at a young age without first having many polyps.

ileostomy: an operation in which the end of the small intestine, the ileum, is attached to an opening in the abdominal wall. The contents of the intestine, unformed stool, are expelled through this opening into a bag called an appliance.

imaging studies: methods used to produce pictures of internal body structures. Some imaging methods used to help diagnose or stage cancer are x-rays, CT scans, magnetic resonance imaging (MRI), and ultrasound.

immune system: the complex system by which the body resists infection by germs such as bacteria or viruses and rejects transplanted tissues or organs. The immune system may also help the body fight some cancers.

incidence: the number of new cases of a disease that occur in a population each year. Compare to prevalence.

incision: a cut made during surgery.

inflammatory bowel disease: a chronic condition (either ulcerative colitis or Crohn's disease) in which the colon is inflamed over a long period of time and may have ulcers in its lining, and which increases a person's risk of colorectal cancer.

internal radiation: treatment involving implantation of a radioactive substance; see brachytherapy.

interstitial radiation therapy: a type of internal radiation or brachytherapy treatment in which a radioactive implant is placed directly into the tissue (not in a body cavity).

intestines: the part of the digestive tract from the end of the stomach (pylorus) to the anus, which absorbs nutrients and water from food into the bloodstream. It includes the small intestine and the large intestine.

intravenous (IV): a method of supplying fluids and medications using a needle inserted in a vein.

invasive cancer: cancer that has spread beyond the layer of cells where it first developed to involve nearby tissues.

investigational: under study; often used to describe drugs used in clinical trials that are not yet available to the general public.

laparoscope: a long, slender tube inserted into the abdomen through a very small incision. Surgeons with experience in laparoscopy can do some types of surgery for colorectal cancer using special surgical instruments operated through the laparoscope.

laparoscopy: examination of the abdominal cavity with an instrument called a laparoscope.

large intestine: *see* **colon**.

local anesthesia: *see* **anesthesia**.

local recurrence: *see* **recurrence**.

lower GI series: series of x-rays of the intestines taken after a barium enema is given.

lymphadenectomy: surgical removal of lymph nodes. After removal, the lymph nodes are examined by microscope to see if cancer has spread. Also called lymph node dissection.

lymphatic system: the tissues and organs (including lymph nodes, spleen, thymus, and bone marrow) that produce and store lymphocytes (cells that fight infection) and the channels that carry the lymph fluid. The entire lymphatic system is an important part of the body's immune system. Invasive cancers sometimes penetrate the lymphatic vessels (channels) and spread (metastasize) to lymph nodes.

lymph: clear fluid that flows through the lymphatic vessels and contains cells known as lymphocytes. These cells are important in fighting infections and may also have a role in fighting cancer.

lymph nodes: small bean-shaped collections of immune system tissue such as lymphocytes, found along lymphatic vessels. They remove cell waste and fluids from lymph. They help fight infections and also have a role in fighting cancer, although cancers sometimes spread through them. Also called **lymph glands**.

lymphocytes: a type of white blood cell that helps the body fight infection.

lymphoma: cancer of a type of white blood cells called lymphocytes. Lymphoma usually starts in lymph nodes, but less often can develop in organs of the digestive system.

magnetic resonance imaging (MRI): a method of taking pictures of the inside of the body. Instead of using x-rays, MRI uses a powerful magnet to send radio waves through the body. The images appear on a computer screen as well as on film. Like x-rays, the procedure is physically painless, but some people may feel confined inside the MRI machine.

malignant tumor: a mass of cancer cells that may invade surrounding tissues or spread (metastasize) to distant areas of the body.

margin, surgical: the edge of a sample removed during surgery. A negative surgical margin is a sign that no cancer was left behind. A positive surgical margin indicates that cancer cells are found at the outer edge of the removed sample and is usually a sign that some cancer remains in the body.

medical oncologist: a doctor who is specially trained to diagnose cancer and treat it with chemotherapy and other drugs.

metastasis: the spread of cancer cells to distant areas of the body by way of the lymph system or bloodstream.

mucinous carcinoma: a type of adenocarcinoma that is formed by cancer cells that produce large amounts of mucus.

mucosa: mucous membrane; the innermost lining layer of the colon and rectum.

mucus: the thick fluid secreted by mucous membranes and glands.

negative margin: *see* **margin**.

neoadjuvant therapy: treatment given before the main treatment. Compare to **adjuvant therapy**.

neoplasm: an abnormal growth (tumor) that starts from a single altered cell; a neoplasm may be benign or malignant. Cancer is a malignant neoplasm.

node: lymph node; *see* **lymphatic system**.

nodal status: indicates whether the cancer has spread (node-positive) or has not spread (node-negative) to lymph nodes.

nurse practitioner: a registered nurse with a master's or doctoral degree. Licensed nurse practitioners diagnose and manage illness and disease, usually working closely with a doctor. In many states, they may prescribe medications.

oncogenes: genes that promote cell growth and multiplication. These genes are normally present in all cells. But oncogenes may undergo changes that activate them, causing cells to grow too quickly and form tumors.

oncologist: a doctor with special training in the diagnosis and treatment of cancer.

oncology: the branch of medicine concerned with the diagnosis and treatment of cancer.

oncology clinical nurse specialist: a registered nurse with a master's degree in oncology who specializes in the care of cancer patients. Oncology nurse specialists may prepare and administer treatments, monitor patients, prescribe and provide supportive care, and teach and counsel patients and their families.

oncology social worker: a person with a master's degree in social work who is an expert in coordinating and providing non-medical care to patients. The oncology social worker provides counseling and assistance to people with cancer and their families, especially in dealing with the non-medical issues that can result from cancer, such as financial problems, housing (when treatments must be taken at a facility away from home), and child care.

palliative treatment: therapy that relieves symptoms, such as pain or blockage of urine flow, but is not expected to cure the cancer. Its main purpose is to improve the patient's quality of life.

pancolitis: ulcerative colitis that involves the entire colon.

pathologist: a doctor who specializes in diagnosis and classification of diseases by lab tests such as examining cells under a microscope. The pathologist determines whether a tumor is benign or cancerous, and if cancerous the exact cell type and grade.

permanent section: a method of preparing tissue for microscopic examination. The tissue is soaked in formaldehyde, processed in various chemicals, surrounded by a block of wax, sliced very thin, attached to a microscope slide and stained. This usually takes 1-2 days. It provides a clear view of the sample so that the presence or absence of cancer can be determined.

platelet: a part of the blood that plugs up holes in blood vessels after an injury. Chemotherapy can cause a drop in the platelet count, a condition called thrombocytopenia that carries risk of excessive bleeding.

polyp: a growth from a mucous membrane commonly found in organs such as the rectum, the colon, or other organs. Some polyps may be precancerous or may contain cancer cells.

polypectomy: surgery to remove a polyp.

positive margin: *see* **margin**.

prevalence: a measure of the proportion of persons in the population with a particular disease at a given time. Compare with incidence.

primary site: the place where cancer begins. Primary cancer is usually named after the organ in which it starts. For example, cancer that starts in the colon is always colon cancer even if it spreads (metastasizes) to other organs such as the liver.

primary treatment: the first, and usually the most important, treatment.

prognosis: a prediction of the course of disease; the outlook for the chances of survival.

protocol: a formal outline or plan, such as a description of what treatments a patient will receive and exactly when each should be given. *See also*, **regimen**.

rad: stands for "radiation absorbed dose," a measurement of the amount of radiation absorbed by the body. The term rad is being replaced by cGy. *See* **cGy**.

radiation oncologist: a doctor who specializes in using radiation to treat cancer.

radiation proctitis: a possible side effect of radiation therapy, involving inflammation of the rectum and anus. Problems can include pain, bowel frequency, bowel urgency, bleeding, chronic burning, or rectal leakage.

radiation therapy: treatment with high-energy rays (such as x-rays) to kill or shrink cancer cells. The radiation may come from outside of the body (external radiation) or from radioactive materials placed directly in the tumor (brachytherapy or internal radiation). Radiation therapy may be used as the main treatment for a cancer, to reduce the size of a cancer before surgery, or to destroy any remaining cancer cells after surgery. In advanced cancer cases, it may also be used as palliative treatment.

radiologist: a doctor with special training in diagnosis of diseases by interpreting x-rays and other types of diagnostic imaging studies; for example, CT and MRI scans.

rectum: the lower part of the large intestine, just above the anus.

recurrence: the return of cancer after treatment. Local recurrence means that the cancer has come back at the same place as the original cancer. Regional recurrence means that the cancer has come back after treatment in the lymph nodes near the primary site. Distant recurrence is when cancer metastasizes after treatment to distant organs or tissues (such as the lungs, liver, bone marrow, or brain).

red blood cells: blood cells that contain hemoglobin, the substance that carries oxygen to all of the cells of the body.

refractory: no longer responsive to a certain therapy.

regimen: a strict, regulated plan (such as diet, exercise, or other activity) designed to reach certain goals. In cancer treatment, a plan to treat cancer. *See also*, **protocol**.

regional involvement: the spread of cancer from its original site to nearby areas such as lymph nodes, but not to distant sites.

regression: reduction of the size of the tumor or the extent of the cancer.

rehabilitation: activities to help a person adjust, heal, and return to as full and productive a life as possible after injury or illness. This may involve physical restoration (such as the use of prostheses, exercises, and physical therapy), counseling, and emotional support.

relapse: reappearance of cancer after a disease-free period. *See also*, **recurrence**.

remission: complete or partial disappearance of the signs and symptoms of cancer in response to treatment; the period during which a disease is under control. A remission may not be a cure.

risk factor: anything that affects a person's chance of getting a disease such as cancer. Different cancers have different risk factors. For example, unprotected exposure to strong sunlight is a risk factor for skin cancer; smoking is a risk factor for lung, mouth, larynx, and other cancers. Some risk factors, such as smoking, can be controlled. Others, like a person's age, can't be changed.

screening: the search for disease, such as cancer, in people without symptoms. For example, screening measures recommended by the American Cancer Society for colorectal cancer include one of the following: flexible sigmoidoscopy; fecal occult blood test; flexible sigmoidoscopy plus fecal occult blood test; colonoscopy; or double contrast barium enema. Screening may also refer to coordinated programs in large populations.

segmental resection: surgery in which the cancer and a length of normal colon on either side of the cancer as well as the nearby lymph nodes are removed. The remaining sections of the colon are then attached back together.

side effects: unwanted effects of treatment, such as hair loss caused by chemotherapy and fatigue caused by radiation therapy.

sigmoid colon: the fourth section of the colon. It is known as the sigmoid colon because of its S-shape. The sigmoid colon attaches to the rectum, which in turn connects to the anus, the opening where waste matter passes out of the body.

sigmoidoscope (flexible): a slender, flexible, hollow, lighted tube about the thickness of a finger. It is inserted through the rectum up into the colon during a flexible sigmoidoscopy. This allows the doctor to look at the inside of the rectum and part of the colon for cancer or for polyps. The sigmoidoscope is connected to a video camera and video display monitor so the doctor can look closely at the inside of your colon. This test may be some-what uncomfortable, but it should not be painful.

sign: an observable physical change caused by an illness. Compare to **symptom**.

simulation: a process involving special x-ray pictures that are used to plan radiation treatment so that the area to be treated is precisely located and marked for treatment.

small intestine: the longest section of the GI tract. It breaks down food and absorbs most of the nutrients. The small intestine leads into the colon. Also called the small bowel.

staging: the process of finding out whether cancer has spread and if so, how far. There is more than one system for staging colorectal cancer, including the AJCC/TNM, Dukes, and Astler-Coller systems.

The TNM system, which is used most often, gives 3 key pieces of information:
- **T** refers to the size of the **t**umor
- **N** describes how far the cancer has spread to near-by lymph **n**odes
- **M** shows whether the cancer has spread (**m**etastasized) to other organs of the body

Letters or numbers after the T, N, and M give more details about each of these factors. To make this information clearer, the TNM descriptions can be grouped together into a simpler set of stages, labeled with Roman numerals (usually from I to IV). In general, the lower the number, the less the cancer has spread. A higher number means a more serious cancer.

The 2 types of staging are:
- **clinical staging:** an estimate of the extent of cancer based on physical exam, biopsy results, and imaging tests.
- **pathologic staging:** an estimate of the extent of cancer by direct study of the samples removed during surgery.

standard therapy: the most commonly used and widely accepted form of treatment for a disease.

stool: solid waste matter; feces.

symptom: a change in the body caused by an illness, as described by the person experiencing it. Compare to **sign**.

systemic therapy: treatment that reaches and affects cells throughout the body; for example, chemotherapy.

TNM: *see* **staging**.

therapy: any of the measures taken to treat a disease. *See also* **standard therapy**, **alternative therapy**, **complementary therapy**, and **unproven therapy**.

tissue: a collection of cells, united to perform a common function in the body.

total colon exam (TCE): an exam that looks at the entire large intestine, such as colonoscopy or double contrast barium enema.

transverse colon: the second section of the colon. It is called the transverse colon because it goes across the body from the right to the left side.

tumor: an abnormal lump or mass of tissue. Tumors can be benign (not cancerous) or malignant (cancerous).

tumor suppressor genes: genes that slow down cell division or cause cells to die at the appropriate time. Changes that inactivate these genes can lead to too much cell growth and development of cancer.

ulcerative colitis: a type of inflammatory bowel disease. In this condition, the colon is inflamed over a long period of time. This increases a person's risk of developing colon cancer, so starting colorectal cancer screening earlier and doing these tests more often is recommended.

unproven therapy: any therapy that has not been scientifically tested and approved.

virtual colonoscopy: examination of the colon for polyps using special computerized tomography (CT) scans. The images are combined by a computer to create a 3D model of the colon, which doctors can "fly through" on a computer screen. It is not yet clear if this new technique is as effective as other screening methods for colon cancer.

white blood cells: cells that help defend the body against infections. There are several types of white blood cells. Certain cancer treatments such as chemotherapy can reduce the number of these cells and make a person more likely to get infections.

x-ray: one form of radiation that can be used at low levels to produce an image of the body on film or at high levels to destroy cancer cells.

Index